TRUTHFULNESS AND TRAGEDY

Truthfulness and Tragedy

Further Investigations in Christian Ethics

Stanley Hauerwas

with

Richard Bondi and David B. Burrell

UNIVERSITY OF NOTRE DAME PRESS

NOTRE DAME   LONDON

Library of Congress Cataloging in Publication Data

Hauerwas, Stanley, 1940–
  Truthfulness and tragedy.

  Includes bibliographical references and index.
  1. Christian ethics—Addresses, essays,
lectures. 2. Social ethics—Addresses, essays,
lectures. I. Bondi, Richard, joint author.
II. Burrell, David B., joint author. III. Title.
BJ1251.H33   241   76-30425
ISBN 0-268-01831-6
ISBN 0-268-01832-4 pbk.

To
John Score,
Friend and Teacher

We would rather be ruined than changed,
We would rather die in our dread
Than Climb the Cross of the moment
And see our illusions die.

W. H. Auden

There is a law in me or in my mind, the law of my integrity;
and there are many laws in my members, the laws of response
to many systems of action about me.

H. R. Niebuhr

Man's biological survival is intimately bound up with, but
subordinate to, his awareness of the truth of things.

K. O. L. Burridge

Contents

Contents

PART THREE

Children, Suffering
and the Skill to Care

Preface

David Burrell and Richard Bondi are listed as contributing authors to this volume because without them these essays would not have been possible. Father Burrell is the joint author of two of the essays, Mr. Bondi of another.

But beyond their direct contribution I owe them much more. Mr. Bondi has read, criticized and edited almost every essay in this book. He has never failed to make valuable suggestions which have improved the quality of the work. Father Burrell has also read and criticized many of these essays. Yet beyond that, many of the ideas and arguments presented here are as much or more his than mine. Together with Sister Elena Malits, we have taught a course called Story and Theology for the last four years. Through the process I am sure many of the ideas I think are "mine" are more ours than I even suspect.

Moreover, I wish to thank all those at the University of Notre Dame who have helped me directly and indirectly. I am sure that this book would have been impossible without the context this university provides for serious intellectual work and theological reflection. I suspect that few universities have better departmental interaction. Moreover, the moral and religious life of those who live and work at Notre Dame has been equally—if not more—important for me as the intellectual opportunity.

Special thanks are due to my colleagues in the Department of Theology. The high level of critical and constructive reflection they engender has been invaluable for my own work. It is my hope that we are developing at Notre Dame a theological style that can make a contribution to the theological task. Certainly there is no one position that characterizes our department, but there is a commitment to do serious theological reflection within the Christian and Jewish traditions. At the very least this means that the question of the truth of religious convictions can be bracketed by no discipline—whether it be the study of scripture, Judaism, Patristics, liturgy or ethics. It is our hope that the attempt to take seriously the claims of the tradition represented by Notre Dame will at least serve to break the stranglehold of the academic orthodoxy as it is enshrined in our current scholarly "areas." How interesting any intellectual work is depends, finally, on courage as much as scholarship. At

Notre Dame we are trying to do theology in a manner that reflects the courage of our convictions.

The academic respectability of theology will not be secured by trying to make theology as uninteresting as sociology or by taking refuge in the "study of" methodology. Rather, theology is appropriately done in the university when it is done in a manner that makes clear that it deals with matters of human significance. Moreover, it is only when we take our own tradition seriously that we can feel the pain caused, and recognize the conceptual issues raised by those who do not share our convictions. That is why, for example, we are committed at Notre Dame to take seriously the implications for Christian theology of the continued existence and vitality of the people of God, i.e., the Jews.

I am a Christian theologian and ethicist because I find myself deeply held by the convictions that Christians hold about the nature of God, Christ and human existence. But even if I were not so convinced, I would consider it academically misleading to think that theology could be done apart from a tradition. We must constantly relearn the lesson that truth does not come through trying to assume a universal or neutral point of view, but through the struggle to live truthfully in relation to a particular tradition. I owe Notre Dame so much because I have found here people who carry on that struggle. I am sure such people exist everywhere; I found them here.

There are many people I need to thank, but I cannot list them all. There are some, however, I cannot pass over, since without their friendship I do not think this work could have been done. Therefore, I acknowledge a special debt to Peri and Beverly Arnold, Mary Jo Weaver, and, of course, to Anne and Adam.

Acknowledgments

The author and publisher are grateful to the following for permission to reprint:

Institute of Society, Ethics and the Life Sciences, Hastings-on-Hudson, N.Y., for "From System to Story: An Alternative Pattern for Rationality in Ethics," published in H. Tristram Engelhardt, Jr., and Daniel Callahan (eds.), *Knowledge, Value and Belief,* vol. II of the Foundations of Ethics and Its Relationship to Science, 1977;

Journal of Religious Ethics, 3 (Spring 1975), for "Obligation and Virtue Once More";

American Journal of Jurisprudence, 20 (1975), for "Natural Law, Tragedy, and Theological Ethics";

Religion in Life, Autumn, 1976, for "Story and Theology";

Journal of Religious Ethics, 2 (May 1974), for "Self-Deception and Autobiography: Theology and Ethical Reflections on Spear's *Inside the Third Reich*";

Journal of the American Academy of Religion, 44, 3 (September 1976), for "Memory, Community, and the Reasons for Living: Theological and Ethical Reflections on Suicide and Euthanasia";

Thought, 49, 194 (September 1974), for "The Moral Limits of Population Control";

Connecticut Medicine, 39, 12 (December 1975) for "Must a Patient Be a Person to be a Patient, or My Uncle Charlie Is Not Much of a Person But He Is Still My Uncle Charlie";

Interpretation, Spring, 1977, for "Politics of Charity";

Pastoral Ministry to the Handicapped (*National Apostolate for the Mentally Retarded Quarterly Publication,* 6, 3 [Fall, 1975]), for "Having and Learning How to Care for Retarded Children";

The Linacre Quarterly, 40, 4 (November 1973), for "The Retarded and Criteria for the Human";

The American Journal of the Medical Sciences, 269, 2 (March-April 1975), for "The Demands and Limits of Care: Ethical Reflections on the Moral Dilemmas of Neonatal Intensive Care."

Introduction

1. The Purpose of This Book

I have brought these essays together because they extend and help clarify the position I began in *Character and the Christian Life* and *Vision and Virtue*. The justification for collecting the essays in one book is that taken together they represent a position the strength or weakness of which is not so evident in the individual essays. Whether the position will be judged more or less adequate, I can at least claim that it challenges some of the dominant paradigms currently shared by philosophical and theological ethicists. It is my hunch that part of the reason that Christian ethics is seldom read by anyone other than those working in the area is not that what ethicists say is wrong, but that it is just uninteresting. I hope these essays are at least interesting insofar as they demonstrate that Christians make serious claims about the moral life that anyone intent on living seriously should not ignore.

Even though these essays seem to cover a wide range of topics, each one has been conceived to further a central project. I have no interest in providing a "system" or "foundation" for Christian ethics, but I do have a set of systematic interests—an attempt to provide an account of moral existence and ethical rationality that may help to render the convictions of Christians morally intelligible. More positively, I am trying to do theology in a manner appropriate to the way Christian convictions operate, or should operate, to form and direct lives. By so doing I hope to show that we can have a better idea of what it might mean to say that such convictions are true or false.

1.1 Misconceptions of the Project

These essays should help to make clear that my interest is not just to develop an ethics of virtue or character. Rather, I have employed the concept of character in order to develop the full dimension of a classical Aristotelian

1

conception of ethics. To emphasize the importance of character is not only a way of re-emphasizing the agent's perspective, but also an attempt to rethink what moral objectivity involves. I am not, therefore, trying to supplement the Kantian paradigm that appears to many today to be the only intelligible form of moral objectivity; rather I am trying to provide a new way to conceive of moral rationality and objectivity. It is not the demand for "objective moral judgments" that has misled us, but rather the theories of "objectivity" that have dominated the modern period.

Nowhere is the dominance of the formalist appeal in ethics more apparent than in the interpretations some have brought to arguments like mine. At best, work like mine is considered an interesting overlay to a "real ethics" that tries to provide a formal account of moral objectivity. Or at worst the position is interpreted as a dangerous reassertion of relativism or subjectivism.[1] But the charge of relativism is dependent on the assumption that moral reflection is only secured by providing a knockdown argument against relativism. Rather, following the suggestion of Bernard Williams, I am content to challenge the relativist or subjectivist to try to live out the implications of his position—after all, practical arguments may be best in a practical discipline.[2]

Nor is my emphasis on character an attempt to stress the importance of individual morality as opposed to social concerns. Indeed, I tried to make clear in *Character and the Christian Life* that an individual's character is only intelligible as it draws its substance from a social context. The emphasis on character is, however, an attempt to reconceive how liberal societies and the ethical theories that presuppose them construe the distinction between individual and social. The power of the liberal paradigm in this respect is amply illustrated by the widespread assumption that the distinction between individual and social morality makes sense.

In contrast, I assume that all moral behavior is social, though not all of it need be public. For social reasons we may have areas of our lives kept free from public scrutiny; for public reasons, such areas are thought to be the proper province of the personal. But "the personal" is a social construction, marked off in order to provide for the development of intimacy and the self.

Moreover, societal concern for conformity to certain norms emphasizes conformity rather than the reasons or character of the agent who conforms. Societies rightly regard with indifference the reasons why we do much that we do. The difficulty arises only when moral philosophers assume that the public point of view is the moral point of view. Then ethics becomes minimalistic, concerning itself only with what we ought to do, not with what it would be good to do and for what reasons. No society can long endure as a good society while asking only conformity and not the accompanying virtues.

1.2   The Style of the Essays

Even though these essays appear to be wide-ranging, each has been conceived to develop or illustrate my concern to articulate how Christian convictions form lives. I find the essay a congenial form in that it allows me to double back and pick up what was insufficiently developed in other essays. For example, "Self-Deception and Autobiography" is the earliest essay included in the first section. Even though I think it remains the best essay in the book, I felt that the use of "story" in it was too cryptic. I, therefore, wrote "Story and Theology" in an attempt to make clear what "story" involved and why it is so important for theological concerns. Further, "From System to Story" tries to spell out the ramifications which a focus on story offers for setting canons of rationality in ethics.

I cannot pretend that this way of proceeding has answered all the objections or clarified all the unclarities about my position, but it at least lets me write as though each essay is part of a conversation. For I depend on those readers who read or hear the essay and tell me what remains unclear or just seems wrong. I am then able to revise or write something else that attempts to clarify or to meet the objection. The essay has its limits, but it seems the best form for a still-developing theological ethic.

In this respect it is perhaps worth remarking on the different styles of essays found here. Some have suggested that my work appears as if it were written by two different people. They do not see how the technical, analytic essay such as "Natural Law, Tragedy, and Theological Ethics" can have been written by the same person who wrote the more homelitical "Having and Learning How to Care for Retarded Children." I cannot deny the difference in style, and even though I think that there is a deep unity between those essays, the reason they appear so different is important for understanding much of ethics and theology being done today.

A natural, but mistaken, way of construing the differences would be to speculate that some of this work is academic and other is more popular. But footnotes and analytic style do not make an article intellectually respectable. Only the substance of the thesis and how cogently it is presented constitute a claim to command the attention of serious people. On such grounds, "Having and Learning to Care for Retarded Children" is as serious as any article in this book.

The difference between the styles of the essays is not academic versus popular, but rather direct versus indirect. Much of the work is indirect in the sense that I am trying to make my position intelligible by exposing the strengths and weaknesses of contemporary ethics. For example, even though I find most of the questions raised in the religion-morality discussion misplaced, I try to take the problem seriously in order to show how the questions are occasioned by a mistaken account of ethics. If I did not take the time to develop these kinds of arguments then the systematic significance of a more direct essay such as "Having and Learning..." would not be appreciated.

Likewise, the important systematic point of "Having and Learning..." is that ethically not much can be said about the condition under which retarded children can be welcomed into the world unless one is able to presuppose certain assumptions about parenting—i.e., we must have some idea why we are having children in the first place. The reasons that form our having or not having children are therefore an indication of our most basic convictions. But from the perspective of much of contemporary ethics, to insert that sense of parenting into ethical analysis is to base one's position on an irrational standard. Thus the kind and style of argument I develop in "Having and Learning..." is possible only if the more analytic arguments in the first section of the book make sense. Many will find the first section of the book the harder and less interesting, but without the work done there the essays in the latter half of the book could not have been written. For if theological ethics is ever to be more than slogans—whether "liberation," "redemption" or some other—it must be grounded on arguments.

Another form of indirect argument is found in the essays "The Demands and Limits of Care," "Suffering, Medical Ethics..., " "Moral Limits of Population Control" and "Must a Patient Be a Person...." In each of these essays, in different ways, I try to take the issues as described by the standard account and show how such descriptions involve us in absurdities or counter-intuitive conclusions. My aim in an essay such as "The Demands and Limits of Care" is to show that we cannot make headway on these troubling issues just by trying to determine whether newborns are or are not "persons" and thus capable of bearing "rights." It is my hope that having finished "The Demands and Limits of Care," one might be encouraged to reread "Having and Learning..." with changed appreciation of its systematic significance.

1.3   The Interrelation of the Essays

I have indicated how some of these essays interrelate, but their interrelation is even more complex than I have said. The individual essays do not pick up just one theme from the other essays, but several. Because of this, the essays could have been arranged in several different ways. As the essays now appear, I have tried to group those with a more strictly methodological focus in the first part. "From System to Story" and "Obligation and Virtue Once More" are primarily critical responses to the dominant paradigm which I simply call "the standard account."

The latter essay is a critique of Frankena's account of the relation of obligation and virtue. I have included it, as it helps illustrate in a concrete manner some of the problems characteristic of ethics done in the style of the standard account. Moreover, the wide appeal of Dr. Frankena's excellent introductory text, *Ethics,* makes it important to try to show that his judicious presentation of contemporary "ethics" represents the working out of a particular account of moral rationality within the context of a scholastic tradition. Moreover, Dr. Frankena's honesty, nuanced position and moral concern make criticism of his position particularly important. In that regard I must urge the reader to look at Dr. Frankena's response to my essay in order to see in what ways he thinks I have misinterpreted his position or what unclarities or errors are present in my arguments.[3]

"Natural Law, Tragedy, and Theological Ethics" is a transition essay in the first section in that it sets the contexts for the presentation of my more constructive claims. In an interesting way, traditional formulations of natural law functioned in a manner similar to the standard account to distort the nature of Christian ethics. Natural law's emphasis on rationality as the mark of man tended to separate and give an independence to the natural virtues despite Aquinas' argument that it was possible to distinguish the natural from the supernatural virtues only for intellectual purposes. By trying to reinterpret natural law in terms of the language of virtues—which I think is actually closer to Aquinas' own position—I am suggesting that it is a mistake to offer any one characteristic of man in order to give a center or integrity to the self. What we require is not one overriding "virtue," but a narrative that will provide a direction for our character that is appropriate to the tragic aspect of our existence. The charity that according to Aquinas forms the virtues is nothing less than learning to imitate the God we have found in the life and death of Jesus Christ.

By employing the language of roles I have attempted to show the existential significance of these theoretical issues. One of the major characteristics of our life today is how roles we embody compete for our loyalties. Indeed we tend to think of ourselves as a bundle of roles and we fear there is no self separate from our roles. This condition often tempts us to identify too completely with one role, for it is indeed better to be something rather than nothing. The consequences of such identification can range from unwarranted claims of not being responsible for non-role-related aspects of our existence, to destructive forms of self-deception. I have tried to show that the need to have a sense of self that gives a critical perspective to our roles is correlative to the self being formed by a truthful narrative.

The second part, "Survival, Community, and the Demand for Truthfulness," includes essays that address more directly the substantive issues: limits of the value of survival and the kind of community in which truthfulness can be a way of life. Though these essays are not as explicitly methodological as those in the first section, I hope that the reader will nevertheless see that they are methodologically informed. For example, the somewhat lighthearted "Must a Patient Be a Person To Be A Patient..." involves an attempt to remind us of the oddity and abstractness of the language of "person," a language that the standard account encourages, since it wishes to base what we ought to do on what would pertain between those who know one another only as strangers. According to the standard account, what we owe one another is what we share as "persons," namely rationality. In the paper on suicide and euthanasia I try to show, with Richard Bondi, the implications of seeing one another as "gifts" rather than strangers.

In the "Politics of Charity" I try to spell out how the Christian story should form a community that provides the skills to so regard one another. Such a community should not confuse claims of autonomy with the respect each person has as a creature of God. Rather the church must stand against those who make exaggerated claims to control history in the name of the "freedom of the individual" or the "survival of the species." For the church has been formed by a God who gives us the confidence that each can be trusted as God's gift. The reason suicide is unthinkable in a community formed by such a story is that it denotes a failure to be a community of trust.

Involved in these claims are strong assumptions about the relation of church and world and the nature and content of political theory, each of which needs more argument than can be given here. In brief, my political claims are best exemplified by Richard Adams's portrayal of Hazel's warren in *Watership Down*.[4] For what makes Hazel's warren good, in comparison to the others pictured in the book, is the rabbits' willingness to be a community formed by the stories that have given them the skills and confidence to make use of luck. In such a community the diversity of gifts is welcomed because the narrative that gave direction to the community also provided a sense of equality that encouraged differences. Of course Adams's *Watership Down* is not political theory, but it at least gives an indication of the kind of concerns with which I think political theory must begin to deal. That, however, is a task for another book.

In this book I hope simply to remind us that matters as common as our willingness to have children are important for the nature of social and political community. Once this is understood the question of the relation of church and society can be seen in a new light. To be sure, the people of the church do have a responsibility to the societies in which they dwell, but their first responsibility is to embody their story in a manner that witnesses to the necessity that all men face the limits of this world with joy, good humor, and enthusiasm.

Each of the essays in the final section deals with the problem of how to care for retarded children and the implication of that care for the ethos that should guide medicine. It is my hope that these essays exhibit concretely the implications of my methodological and substantial concerns. I remain convinced that morally no question tells us more about our commitments than "Why should we have children and how should we care for them?" I am not, for heaven's sake, trying to argue that only Christians or Jews have good reasons for having children, but only that their reasons for having children should make a difference in how they regard those born retarded. Other cases deserve separate investigation.

This final section also develops the theme of suffering as a crucial category for understanding Christian ethics. H. Richard Niebuhr observed in *The Responsible Self* that suffering is a subject neglected by academic ethical theory and theological ethics, even though it is obviously present in each of our lives. Moreover, Niebuhr argues that suffering cannot be adequately accounted for from within the spheres of teleological or deontological ethics because

> suffering is the exhibition of the presence in our existence of that which is not under our control, or of the intrusion into our self-legislating existence of an activity operating under another law than ours. Yet it is in the response to suffering that many and perhaps all men, individually and in their groups, define themselves, take on character, develop their ethos. And their responses are functions of their interpretation of what is happening to them as well as of the actions upon them. It is unnecessary to multiply illustrations from history and experience of the actuality and relevance of the approach to man's self-conduct that begins with neither purposes nor laws, but with responses; that begins with the question, not about the self as it is in itself, but as it is in its response-relations to what is given with it and to it. This question is already implied, for example, in the primordial action of parental guidance: "What is the fitting thing? What is going on in the life of the child?"[5]

Also, in the last section I have tried to spell out Niebuhr's suggestion that the willingness to open ourselves to children sets the context for basic issues of our moral existence. Moreover, I try to suggest that the narrative that sets the interpretation of what Christians are doing when they have children provides the skills for welcoming into the world those not "normal." But I hope it is clear that this particular issue is but one aspect of how the Christian character is set through how we are trained to regard suffering.

The final essay, "Medicine as a Tragic Profession" develops themes from all three parts of the book. In it I attempt to show that we cannot and should not expect medicine in itself to provide answers to problems such as how to care for retarded children. To know how to approach these problems we need a practice of medicine formed by a community that has the skills to deal with the tragic. To try to use medicine as means to hide or eradicate the tragic from our lives only makes us less able to deal truthfully with the limits of our existence.

2. The Central Themes

Two obvious interests that I do not want overemphasized are the use of the category of story and the work done here in "medical ethics." I have found the concept of story, or perhaps better, narrative, to be a suggestive way to spell out the substantive content of character. But I also try to use the language of "story" in a carefully controlled sense. I am not trying to do "story theology" or "theology of story," as if this represented some new theological position. Rather I am convinced that narrative is a perennial category for understanding better how the grammar of religious convictions is displayed and how the self is formed by those convictions.

Nor am I interested in developing or providing the basis for medical ethics understood as a distinctive area. It is not by accident that medicine offers a fruitful and rich context for moral reflection. Medicine has always been a moral art even if the development of "scientific medicine" has tended to obscure the moral commitments of medical care. Many are suggesting, rightly I think, that because this has happened medicine today is morally at sea. The ethicist can do little to solve this kind of problem; no discipline of bioethics or medical ethics can replace what only substantive community can provide. But in the meantime, medicine provides a way to remind us how serious it is to confront the dangers present in our life without substantial convictions to guide our way.

There are, however, three central themes that run through this book: (1) the nature of moral rationality and its significance for how theological ethics is conceived; (2) the interdependence of community and truthfulness; and (3) an understanding of the nature of Christian existence. It may help to set the stage for my suggestions concerning these three themes if I indicate the main reason for emphasizing each theme and the interconnection between the themes.

2.1   Rationality and the Christian Narrative

My primary interests are theological. I bear the title "ethicist" only as a way of indicating a set of interests or questions, not as denoting a distinct methodological area. Christian theology is concerned with which theological convictions should be central to the Christian life, and how these convictions might be properly entertained as truthful. It is my hunch that the latter question is not answered by trying to show how theological convictions are rooted in, correlative of, or appropriate to metaphysical or ontological schemes. Rather, the question of truthfulness of our theological convictions is most appropriately raised by asking how through our language and character they form and display our practical affairs. (This does not mean that all metaphysical issues are in all respects unimportant to certain aspects of theological discourse.)

The character that such convictions form is not limited to each individual character, but entails the language, practices and institutions of some community. Therefore, the truthfulness of theological convictions is partly known by the kind of considerations and arguments which their linguistic, liturgical and institutional life fosters. The activity of ethical reflection is not, therefore, one thing that cuts across different communities of discourse, even though certain similarities of form and context may appear. Rather the character of ethical reflection is determined by the convictions and form of the community that calls it forth.

However, most accounts of the nature of ethical rationality have attempted to free reason from the limits of particularistic communities. This has been done by trying to attribute to practical reason the kind of necessity and certitude that Aristotle thought appropriate only to science. But this view of rationality makes it difficult not only to articulate the convictions that inform the Christian life, but also to measure their truthfulness in terms of how they work. In such a model of ethics, Christian conviction cannot help but appear irrelevant or secondary to the central concern of "ethics."

I have therefore tried to develop an account of rationality that does justice to the practical, historical and social nature of moral reason. At the same time, however, I have tried to show that this account of rationality does not imply a vicious relativism or subjectivism. There are "criteria" of moral truthfulness, though such criteria can never be independent of a substantive narrative.

This critique of moral rationality is necessary for my primary concern: articulating the specificity of the Christian moral life. In this respect my criticism of the standard account of moral rationality has close analogies to past critiques of natural law. For past natural law theories have mistakenly encouraged Christian ethics to be done from the bottom up. These theories held that the ethicist should work as far as possible on grounds that everyone shares, using one's theological presuppositions only as a last resort. As a result, the distinctive shape and commitments of the Christian life have been distorted.

Instead, Christian ethics should begin with Christian convictions and how they shape our understanding of moral existence. To begin here is not to deny that all people may share important moral characteristics, but, as I try to show in the essay on natural law, these shared characteristics are not of the sort that allows one to actually anchor morality in them. Many Christians believe that the Christian moral life is true for all people—that the Christian morally struggles with the same concerns others do—but from that conviction it does not follow that all people have come to form their actual moral life in ways familiar to us. The "universality" of our Christian convictions rather gives us the courage to live them out and witness to them in strange and foreign lands—including the U.S.A. It is only when Christians are willing to have their lives formed by the particularity of their convictions and only as they learn to articulate those convictions that they will have an authentic basis for finding what they share in common with those not Christians.

2.2   Truthfulness and Community

This methodological issue is related to the second theme that these essays develop: the necessary connection between truthfulness and community. Community is the necessary condition for truthfulness, but truthfulness is equally necessary for the building of noncoercive community. It is my contention that the relation of church to world is not just an issue for social ethics but rather is crucial for the very concept of moral truthfulness. The limits of community and the narrative that sets its topography constitute the conditions for providing us with the skills to live truthfully.

Moreover, universal community exists only as an eschatological hope. All we know is the particular and limited communities that have formed us and that we have chosen. So, the extent that Christians can make common cause with the societies in which they exist will depend on the nature and shape of those societies. No doctrine of natural law can insure in advance that Christians will find large areas of common agreement with their non-Christian neighbors.

In this respect my attempt to suggest the relation between community and truthfulness also involves a criticism of our contemporary liberal society. For it is my belief that the liberal commitment to the freedom of the individual does not provide an ethos sufficient for the nurturing of morally truthful lives. Moreover, the ethical theory correlative of such societies, namely, the attempt to limit ethics to the obligations incumbent on each other as self-interested units which rationally calculate how best to secure their own survival, is a formula for the disintegration of the moral self. For liberal ethical theory, the only "ethically interesting" concerns are those that are duty-bound, public or legal.

Christians should prefer to exist in societies that allow the free proclamation and practice of the Christian life. Insofar as liberal societies do that we must be thankful, but we must also remember that the "freedom of the individual" is not a sufficient political translation of the "freedom of the gospel" to wider society. There are many forms of society and government that have provided conditions for the practice of our faith. No one of them is sufficient to allow the Christian to assume that his obligation as Christian is identical to the obligations of the society in which he lives.

This does not mean that Christians can reject the ethical demand to be able to give public reasons for their moral behavior. But the more important question is which public constitutes our primary home? My suggestion that the first social, ethical task of the church is to be herself—which draws out the implications of John Howard Yoder's position—is not simply a tactical move. Rather it is the claim that the church's primary mission is to be a community that keeps alive the language and narrative necessary to form lives in a truthful manner.

The church does have a social, ethical responsibility toward wider society, but it is a task that she must fulfill on her own terms. The first task is to be a community that keeps alive the language of the faith through the liturgical, preaching and teaching offices of the community. In other words, the church serves society best by striving to be a community of truthfulness and care. Otherwise, the wider society cannot even know what it means to be the "world."

For example, I suggest in the essay on suicide that the church must be a community that keeps alive the language of gift of life. As a result, suicide should be pejoratively regarded, that is we should continue to describe unjustified self-infliction of death as suicide. I suggest that liberal society has little consistent reason to continue such a description; or if it continues to use the locution "suicide," it distorts the moral life as it encourages the assumption that survival is a central virtue for individual and social existence. The church, by striving to remain a community were "suicide" can be used in a morally accurate manner, thus holds out an alternative to wider society. In like manner I suggest that the church serves society by being a people constituted by their willingness to have children in the face of the terrors of this existence.

It may seem strange to some to speak of these matters as conditions for truthfulness. But if we remember that moral truthfulness cannot be had simply by trying to describe the world, then the need to have a language and narrative appropriate to *our* world is inescapable. But it must be a language that provides us with the skills to face our own and other's deaths without weaving false webs of personal significance.

2.3 Truthfulness and Tragedy

This last point brings me to the final theme that informs these essays, an understanding of the nature of Christian existence. This aspect of my project can be separated from the methodological arguments above, though it is dependent on them. It might well be possible for others to emphasize a different conception of Christian existence while accepting the arguments concerning the nature of rationality and the significance of community. The gospel is too rich for any one account of Christian existence to be adequate. Different conditions serve to remind us of parts of the Christian life we have forgotten. The claims I make in this respect are therefore put forward as but one attempt to remind Christians what kind of life they are committed to living if they believe that their lives are not their own but God's.

My basic thesis here is contained in the title *Truthfulness and Tragedy*, for a truthful narrative is one that gives us the means to accept the tragic without succumbing to self-deceiving explanations. I will perhaps be criticized for failing to define tragedy with more exactness, but my point is different from the literary question of how to distinguish comedy from tragedy. I am suggesting that once it is recognized that survival is not a worthy moral end, then tragedy can be seen not to be just unfortunate events but a necessary characteristic of our lives. As Jean Giraudoux says, "Tragedy is the affirmation of a horrible bond between men and a greater fate than man's fate."

We must be something rather than nothing—a platitude to be sure. But the something we must be is a trade-off against our survival and necessarily the survival of others. All narratives that offer themselves as significant make us and others pay for our adherence to them. We seldom wish to acknowledge this, and we comfort ourselves with the lie that we can live our lives without harming those around us. But we are tied together too intimately for any such illusion to be sustained.

The question is, which narrative gives us the ability to form our existence appropriate to its tragic character? For the Christian, the gospel represents an elaborate training in the appropriation of skills to live joyously in the face of the tragic. For we believe, on the basis of the cross, that our lives are sustained by a God who has taken the tragic into his own life. Since we believe that our home and our significance are in him, we are freed from the obsession of securing our significance against death. We are thus given the time and space that provides the condition for faithfulness.

It is only because God grounds our confidence in his own goodness that we can take the terrible risk of refusing to take up the means of violence to secure relative goods. For our task is not to bring God's kingdom, but rather to witness to it by being the earnest of his kingdom of peace. We are confident that through his calling of Israel, the sending of his Son, and his guidance of the church his kingdom will prevail.

PART ONE

Rationality
and the Christian Story

1. From System to Story:
An Alternative Pattern for
Rationality in Ethics

with David B. Burrell

1. Narrative, Ethics and Theology

In the interest of securing a rational foundation for morality, contemporary ethical theory has ignored or rejected the significance of narrative for ethical reflection. It is our contention that this has been a profound mistake resulting in a distorted account of moral experience. Furthermore, the attempt to portray practical reason independent of narrative contexts has made it difficult to assess the value which convictions characteristic of Christians or Jews might have for moral existence. As a result, we have lost sight of the ways these traditions might help us deal with the moral issues raised by modern science and medicine.[1]

We will develop two independent but interrelated theses in order to illustrate and substantiate these claims. First, we will try to establish the significance of narrative for ethical reflection. By the phrase, "the significance of narrative," we mean to call attention to three points:[2] (1) that character and moral notions only take on meaning in a narrative; (2) that narrative and explanation stand in an intimate relationship, and therefore moral disagreements involve rival histories of explanation; and (3) that the standard account of moral objectivity is the obverse of existentialist ethics, since the latter assumes that the failure to secure moral objectivity implies that all moral judgments must be subjective or arbitrary. Ironically, by restricting the meaning of "rationality" the standard account has unwarrantedly expanded the realm of the irrational. This has led some to the mistaken idea that the only way to be free from the tyranny and manipulative aspect of "reason" is to flee into the "irrational." By showing the way narrative can function as a form of rationality we hope to demonstrate that these represent false alternatives.

Second, we will try to show how the convictions displayed in the Christian story have moral significance. We will call particular attention to the manner

15

in which story teaches us to know and do what is right under definite conditions. For at least one indication of the moral truthfulness of a particular narrative is the way it enables us to recognize the limits of our engagements and yet continue to pursue them.

2. The Standard Account
of Moral Rationality

At least partly under the inspiration of the scientific ideal of objectivity,[3] contemporary ethical theory has tried to secure for moral judgments an objectivity that would free such judgments from the subjective beliefs, wants and stories of the agent who makes them. Just as science tries to insure objectivity by adhering to an explicitly disinterested method, so ethical theory tried to show that moral judgments, insofar as they can be considered true, must be the result of an impersonal rationality. Thus moral judgments, whatever else they may involve, must at least be nonegoistic in the sense that they involve no special pleading from the agent's particular history, community identification or otherwise particular point of view to establish their truthfulness.

Thus the hallmark of contemporary ethical theory, whether in a Kantian or utilitarian mode, has been to free moral behavior from the arbitrary and contingent nature of the agent's beliefs, dispositions and character. Just as science strives to free the experiment from the experimenter, so ethically, if we are to avoid unchecked subjectivism or relativism, it is thought that the moral life must be freed from the peculiarities of agents caught in the limits of their particular histories. Ethical rationality assumes it must take the form of science if it is to have any claim to being objective.[4]

There is an interesting parallel to this development in modern medical theory. Eric Cassell has located a tension between the explanation of a disease proper to science and the diagnosis a clinician makes for a particular patient.[5] The latter is well-described by Tolstoy in *War and Peace:*

> Doctors came to see Natasha, both separately and in consultation. They said a great deal in French, in German, and in Latin. They criticised one another, and prescribed the most diverse remedies for all the diseases they were familiar with. But it never occurred to one of them to make the simple reflection that they could not understand the disease from which Natasha was suffering, as no single disease can be fully understood in a living person; for every living person has his complaints unknown to medicine— not a disease of the lungs, of the kidneys, of the skin, of the heart, and so on, as described in medical books, but a disease that consists of one out of the innumerable combinations of ailments of those organs.[6]

The scientific form of rationality is represented by B. F. Skinner's commentary on this quote. Skinner suggests that Tolstoy was justified in calling every sickness a unique event during his day, but uniqueness no longer stands in the way of the development of the science of medicine since we can now supply the necessary general principles of explanation. Thus happily, according to Skinner, "the intuitive wisdom of the old-style diagnostician has been largely replaced by the analytic procedures of the clinic, just as a scientific analysis of behavior will eventually replace the personal interpretation of unique instances."[7]

Even if we were competent to do so, it would not be relevant to our argument to try to determine whether Tolstoy or Skinner, or some combination of both, describes the kind of explanation most appropriate to medical diagnosis (though our hunch lies with Tolstoy). Rather it is our contention that the tendency of modern ethical theory to find a functional equivalent to Skinner's "scientific analysis" has distorted the nature of practical reason. Ethical objectivity cannot be secured by retreating from narrative, but only by being anchored in those narratives that best direct us toward the good.

Many have tried to free the objectivity of moral reason from narrative by arguing that there are basic moral principles, procedures or points of view to which a person is logically or conceptually committed when engaged in moral action or judgment. This logical feature has been associated with such titles as the categorical imperative, the ideal observer, universalizability or more recently, the original position. Each of these in its own way assumes that reasons, if they are to be morally justified, must take the form of judgments that can and must be made from anyone's point of view.[8] All of the views assume that "objectivity" will be attained in the moral life only by freeing moral judgments from the "subjective" story of the agent.

This tradition has been criticized for the formal nature of its account of moral rationality, i.e., it seems to secure the objectivity of moral judgment exactly by vacating the moral life of all substantive content. Such criticism fails to appreciate, however, that these accounts of moral rationality are attempts to secure a "thin" theory of the moral life in order to provide an account of moral duty that is not subject to any community or tradition. Such theories are not meant to tell us how to be good in relation to some ideal, but rather to insure that what we owe to others as strangers, not as friends or sharers in a tradition, is nonarbitrary.

What I am morally obligated to do is not what derives from being a father, or a son, or an American, or a teacher, or a doctor, or a Christian, but what follows from my being a person constituted by reason. To be sure all these other roles or relations may involve behavior that is good to do, but such behavior cannot be required except as it can be based upon or construed as appropriate to rationality itself. This is usually done by translating such role-dependent obligations as relations of promise-keeping that are universalizable. (Of course, what cannot be given are any moral reasons why I should become a husband, father, teacher, doctor or Christian in the first place.)

It is our contention, however, that the standard account of moral rationality distorts the nature of the moral life by: (1) placing an unwarranted emphasis on particular decisions or quandaries; (2) by failing to account for the significance of moral notions and how they work to provide us skills of perception; and (3) by separating the agent from his interests. We will briefly spell out each of these criticisms and suggest how each stems in part from the way standard accounts avoid acknowledging the narrative character of moral existence.

2.1 Decisions, Character and Narrative

In his article, "Quandary Ethics," Edmund Pincoffs has called attention to the way contemporary ethics concentrates on problems—situations in which it is hard to know what to do—as paradigmatic concerns for moral analysis.[9] On such a model, ethics becomes a decision procedure for resolving conflict-of-choice situations. This model assumes that no one faces an ethical issue until they find themselves in a quandary: should I or should I not have an abortion, etc. Thus the moral life appears to be concerned primarily with "hard decisions."

This picture of the moral life is not accidental, given the standard account of moral rationality. For the assumption that most of our moral concerns are "problems" suggests that ethics can be construed as a rational science that evaluates alternative "solutions." Moral decisions should be based on rationally derived principles that are not relative to any one set of convictions. Ethics becomes a branch of decision theory. Like many of the so-called policy sciences, ethics becomes committed to those descriptions of the moral life that will prove relevant to its mode of analysis, that is, one which sees the moral life consisting of dilemmas open to rational "solutions."

By concentrating on "decisions" about "problems," this kind of ethical analysis gives the impression that judgments can be justified apart from the agent who finds himself or herself in the situation. What matters is not that David Burrell or Stanley Hauerwas confronts a certain quandary, but that anyone may or can confront X or Y. The only intentions or reasons for our behavior that are morally interesting are those that anyone might have. So in considering the question of abortion, questions like Why did the pregnancy occur? What kind of community do you live in? What do you believe about the place of children? may be psychologically interesting but cannot be allowed to enter into the justification of the decision. For such matters are bound to vary from one agent to another. The "personal" can only be morally significant to the extent that it can be translated into the "impersonal."

(Though it is not central to our case, one of the implications of the standard account of rationality is its conservative force. Ethical choice is always making do in the societal framework we inherit, because it is only in such a framework that we are able to have a problem at all. But often the precise problem at issue cannot arise or be articulated given the limits of our society or culture. We suspect that this ineptness betrays a commitment of contemporary ethical theory to political liberalism: one can concentrate on the justification of moral decisions because one accepts the surrounding social order with its moral categories. In this sense modern ethical theory is functionally like modern pluralist democratic theory: it can afford to be concerned with incremental social change, to celebrate "issue" politics, because it assumes the underlying social structures are just.)[10]

By restricting rationality to choices between alternative courses of action, the various normative theories formed in accordance with the standard account have difficulty explaining the moral necessity to choose between lesser evils.[11] Since rational choice is also our moral duty, it must also be a good duty. Otherwise one would be obliged rationally to do what is morally a lesser evil. There is no place for moral tragedy; whatever is morally obligatory must be good, even though the consequences may be less than happy. We may subjectively regret what we had to do, but it cannot be a moral regret. The fact that modern deontological and teleological theories assume that the lesser evil cannot be a moral duty witnesses to their common commitment to the standard view of moral rationality.

The problem of the lesser evil usually refers to tragic choices externally imposed, e.g., the necessity of killing civilians in order to halt the manufacture of weapons. Yet the language of "necessity" is often misleading, for part of the "necessity" is the character of the actors, whether they be individuals or nations. Because moral philosophy under the influence of the standard account has thought it impossible to discuss what kind of character we should have—that, after all, is the result of the accident of birth and psychological conditioning—it has been assumed that moral deliberation must accept the limits of the decision required by his or her character. At best, "character" can be discussed in terms of "moral education"; but since the "moral" in education is determined by the standard account, it does not get us very far in addressing what kind of people we ought to be.

As a result, the standard account simply ignores the fact that most of the convictions that charge us morally are like the air we breathe—we never notice them. We never notice them precisely because they form us not to describe the world in certain ways and not to make certain matters subject to decision. Thus we assume that it is wrong to kill children without good reason. Or even more strongly we assume that it is our duty to provide children (and others who cannot protect themselves) with care that we do not need to give to the stranger. These are not matters that we need to articulate or decide about; their force lies rather in their not being subject to decision. And morally we must have the kind of character that keeps us from subjecting them to decision.

(What makes "medical ethics" so difficult is the penchant of medical care to force decisions that seem to call into question aspects of our life that we assumed not to be matters of decision, e.g., should we provide medical care for children who are born with major disabilities such as meningomyelocele.[12] In this respect, the current interest in "medical ethics" does not simply represent a response to issues arising in modern medicine, but also reflects the penchant of the standard account to respond to dilemmas.)

Another way to make this point is that the standard account, by concentrating on decision, fails to deal adequately with the formation of a moral self, i.e., the virtues and character we think it important for moral agents to acquire. But the kind of decisions we confront, indeed the very way we describe a situation, is a function of the kind of character we have. And character is not acquired through decisions, though it may be confirmed and qualified there; rather, it is acquired through the beliefs and dispositions we have come to possess.

But from the perspective of the standard account, beliefs and dispositions cannot be subject to rational deliberation and formation.[13] Positions based on the standard account do not claim that our dispositions, or our character, are irrelevant to how we act morally. But these aspects of our self are rational only as they enter into a moral decision. It is our contention, however, that it is character, inasmuch as it is displayed by a narrative, that provides the context necessary to pose the terms of a decision, or to determine whether a decision should be made at all.[14]

We cannot account for our moral life solely by the decisions we make; we also need the narrative that forms us to have one kind of character rather than another. These narratives are not arbitrarily acquired, although they will embody many factors we might consider "contingent." As our stories, however, they will determine what kind of moral considerations—that is, what reasons—will count at all. Hence these narratives must be included in any account of moral rationality that does not unwarrantedly exclude large aspects of our moral existence, i.e., moral character.[15]

The standard account cannot help but view a narrative account as a retreat from moral objectivity. For if the individual agent's intentions and motives— in short, the narrative embodied in his or her character—are to have systematic significance for moral judgment, then it seems that we will have to give preference to the agent's interpretation of what he has done. So the dreaded first person singular, which the standard account was meant to purge from moral argument, would be reintroduced. To recall the force of 'I', however, does not imply that we would propose "because I want to" as a moral reason.

The fact is that the first person singular is seldom the assertion of the solitary 'I,' but rather the narrative of that I. It is exactly the category of narrative that helps us to see that we are not forced to choose between some universal standpoint and the subjectivistic appeals to our own experience. For our experiences always come in the form of narratives that can be checked against themselves as well as against others' experiences. I cannot make my behavior mean anything I want it to mean, for I have learned to understand my life from the stories I have learned from others.

The language the agent uses to describe his behavior, to himself and to others, is not uniquely his; it is *ours,* just as the notions we use have meanings that can be checked for appropriate or inappropriate use. But what allows us to check the truthfulness of these accounts of our behavior are the narratives in which our moral notions gain their paradigm uses. An agent cannot make his behavior mean anything he wants, since at the very least it must make sense within his own story, as well as be compatible with the narrative embodied in the language he uses. All our notions are narrative-dependent, including the notion of rationality.

2.2 Moral Notions, Language and Narrative

We can show how our very notion of rationality depends on narrative by noting how the standard account tends to ignore the significance and meaning of moral notions. For the standard account pictures our world as a *given* about which we need to make decisions. So terms like 'murder', 'stealing', 'abortion', although admitted to be evaluative, are nonetheless regarded as descriptive. However, as Julius Kovesi has persuasively argued, our moral notions are not descriptive in the sense that 'yellow' is, but rather describe only as we have purposes for such descriptions.[16] Moral notions, in other words, like many of our non-moral notions (though we are not nearly so sure as the standard account how this distinction should be made) do not merely describe our activity; they also form it. Marx's claim that the point of philosophy should be not to analyze the world but to change it, is not only a directive to ethicists but also an astute observation about the way our grammar displays the moral direction of our lives. For the notions that form our moral perceptions involve skills that require narratives, that is, accounts of their institutional contexts and purposes, which we must know if we are to know how to employ them correctly. In other words, these notions are more like skills of perception which we must learn how to use properly.

The standard account's attempt to separate our moral notions from their narrative context, by trying to ground or derive their meaning from rationality in itself, has made it difficult to explain why moral controversies are so

irresolvable. The standard account, for example, encourages us to assume that
the pro- and anti-abortion advocates mean the same thing by the word 'abortion'. So it is assumed that the moral disagreement between these two sides
must involve a basic moral principle such as "all life is sacred," or be a
matter of fact such as whether the fetus is considered a human life. But this
kind of analysis fails to see that the issue is not one of principle or fact, but
one of perception determined by a history of interpretation.

Pro- and anti-abortion advocates do not communicate on the notion "abortion," since each group holds a different story about the purpose of the
notion. At least so far as "abortion" is concerned, they live in conceptually
different worlds. This fact does not prohibit discussion. But if it takes place, it
cannot begin with the simple question of whether abortion is right or wrong. It
is rather more like an argument between a member of the PLO and an Israeli
about whether an attack on a village is unjustified terrorism. They both know
the same "facts" but the issue turns on the story each holds, and within which
those "facts" are known.

The advocates of the standard account try to train us to ignore the dependence of the meaning and use of notions on their narrative contexts, by
providing a normative theory for the derivation and justification of basic
moral notions. But to be narrative-dependent is not the same as being theory-
dependent, at least in the way that a utilitarian or deontological position would
have us think. What makes abortion right or wrong is not its capacity to work
for or against the greatest good of the greatest number in a certain subclass.
What sets the context for one's moral judgment is rather the stories we hold
about the place of children in our lives, or the connection one deems ought or
ought not to hold between sexuality and procreation, or some other such
account. Deontological or utilitarian theories that try to free moral notions
from their dependence on examples and the narratives that display them prove
to be too monochromatic to account for the variety of our notions and the
histories on which they are dependent.

There can be no normative theory of the moral life that is sufficient to
capture the rich texture of the many moral notions we inherit. What we
actually possess are various and sometimes conflicting stories that provide us
with the skills to use certain moral notions. What we need to develop is the
reflective capacity to analyze those stories, so that we better understand how
they function. It is not theory-building that develops such a capacity so much
as close attention to the ways our distinctive communities tell their stories.
Furthermore, an analysis of this sort carries us to the point of assessing the
worth these moral notions have for directing our life projects and shaping our
stories.

The standard account's project to supply a theory of basic moral principles from which all other principles and actions can be justified or derived represents an attempt to make the moral life take on the characteristics of a system. But it is profoundly misleading to think that a rational explanation needs to be given for holding rational beliefs,[17] for to attempt to provide such an account assumes that rationality itself does not depend on narrative. What must be faced, however, is that our lives are not and cannot be subject to such an account, for the consistency necessary for governing our lives is more a matter of integrity than one of principle. The narratives that provide the pattern of integrity cannot be based on principle, nor are they engaging ways of talking about principles. Rather, such narratives are the ones which allow us to determine how our behavior "fits" within our ongoing pattern.[18] To be sure, fittingness cannot have the necessitating form desired by those who want the moral life to have the "firmness" of some sciences, but it can exhibit the rationality of a good story.

2.3 Rationality, Alienation and the Self

The standard account also has the distressing effect of making alienation the central moral virtue. We are moral exactly to the extent that we learn to view our desires, interests and passions as if they could belong to anyone. The moral point of view, whether it is construed in a deontological or teleological manner, requires that we view our own projects and life as if we were outside observers. This can perhaps be seen most vividly in utilitarianism (and interestingly in Rawls' account of the original position) as the utilitarian invites us to assume that perspective toward our projects which will produce the best consequences for anyone's life plan. So the standard account obligates us to regard our life as an observer would.

But paradoxically, what makes our projects valuable to us (as Bernard Williams has argued) is that they are ours. As soon as we take the perspective of the standard account we accept the odd position of viewing our stories as if they were anyone's or at least capable of being lived out by anyone. Thus we are required to alienate ourselves from the projects that make us interested in being anything at all.

The alienation involved in the standard account manifests itself in the different ways the self is understood by modern ethical theory. The self is often pictured as consisting of reason and desire, with the primary function of reason being to control desire. It is further assumed that desire or passion can give no clues to the nature of the good, for the good can only be determined in accordance with "reason." Thus the standard account places us in the odd position of excluding pleasure as an integral aspect of doing the good. The good cannot be the satisfaction of desire, since the morality of reason requires a sharp distinction between universal rules of conduct and the "contingent" appetites of individuals.

Not only are we taught to view our desires in contrast to our reason, but the standard account also separates our present from our past. Morally, the self represents a collection of discontinuous decisions bound together only in the measure they approximate the moral point of view. Our moral capacity thus depends exactly on our ability to view our past in discontinuity with our present. The past is a limit, as it can only prevent us from embodying more fully the new opportunities always guaranteed by the moral point of view. Thus our moral potentiality depends on our being able to alienate ourselves from our past in order to grasp the timelessness of the rationality offered by the standard account.[19]

(In theological terms the alienation of the self is a necessary consequence of sinful pretensions. When the self tries to be more than it was meant to be, it becomes alienated from itself and all its relations are disordered. The view of rationality offered by the standard account is pretentious exactly as it encourages us to try to free ourselves from history. In effect, it offers us the possibility of being like God. Ironically enough, however, this is not the God of the Jews and the Christians since, as we shall see, that God does not will himself to be free from history.)

In fairness, the alienation recommended by the standard account is motivated by the interest of securing moral truthfulness. But it mistakenly assumes that truthfulness is possible only if we judge ourselves and others from the position of complete (or as complete as possible) disinterest. Even if it were possible to assume such a stance, however, it would not provide us with the conditions for truthfulness. For morally there is no neutral story that insures the truthfulness of our particular stories. Moreover, any ethical theory that is sufficiently abstract and universal to claim neutrality would not be able to form character. For it would have deprived itself of the notions and convictions which are the necessary conditions for character. Far from assuring truthfulness, a species of rationality which prizes objectivity to the neglect of particular stories distorts moral reasoning by the way it omits the stories of character formation. If truthfulness (and the selflessness characteristic of moral behavior) is to be found, it will have to occur in and through the stories that tie the contingencies of our life together.

It is not our intention to call into question the significance of disinterestedness for the moral life, but rather to deny that recent accounts of "universality" or the "moral point of view" provide adequate basis for such disinterest. For genuine disinterest reflects a non-interest in the self occasioned by the lure of a greater good or a more beautiful object than we can create or will into existence.[20] In this sense we are not able to choose to conform to the moral point of view, for it is a gift. But as a gift it depends on our self being formed by a narrative that provides the conditions for developing the disinterest required for moral behavior.

2.4 The Standard Account's Story

None of the criticisms above constitutes a decisive objection to the standard account, but taken together they indicate that the standard account is seriously inadequate as a description of our moral existence. How then are we to account for the continued dominance of the standard account for contemporary ethical theory? If our analysis has been right, the explanation should be found in the narrative that provides an apparent cogency for the standard account in spite of its internal and external difficulties.[21]

But it is difficult to identify any one narrative that sets the context for the standard account. For it is not one but many narratives that sustain its plausibility. The form of some of these stories is of recent origin, but we suspect that the basic story underlying the standard account is of more ancient lineage, namely, humankind's quest for certainty in a world of contingency.

It seems inappropriate to attribute such a grand story to the standard account, since one of its attractions is its humility; it does not pretend to address matters of the human condition, for it is only a method. As a method it does not promise truth, only clarity.

Yet the process of acculturating ourselves and others in the use of this method requires a systematic disparaging of narrative. For by teaching us to prefer a "principle" or a "rational" description (just as science prefers a statistical description) to a narrative description, the standard account not only fails to account for the significance of narrative but also sets obstacles to any therapy designed to bring that tendency to light. It thus fails to provide us with the critical skills to know the limits of the narrative which currently has us in its grasp.

The reason for this lack of critical perspective lies in the narrative born of the Enlightenment. The plot was given in capsule by Auguste Comte: first came religion in the form of stories, then philosophy in the form of metaphysical analysis, and then science with its exact methods.[22] The story he tells in outline is set within another elaborated by Hegel, to show us how each of these ages supplanted the other as a refinement in the progressive development of reason. So stories are prescientific, according to the story legitimizing the age which calls itself scientific. Yet if one overlooks that budding contradiction, or fails to spell it out because everyone knows that stories are out of favor anyway, then the subterfuge has been worked and the exit blocked off.

Henceforth, any careful or respectable analysis, especially if it is moral in intent, will strike directly for the problem, leaving the rest for journalists who titillate or novelists who entertain. Serious folk, intent on improving the human condition, will have no time for that (except maybe after hours), for they must focus all available talent and resources on solving the problems in front of them. We all recognize the crude polarities acting here, and know how effectively they function as blinders. It is sufficient for our interests to call attention only to the capacity stories hold for eliciting critical awareness, and how an awareness of story enhances that approach known as scientific by awakening it to its presuppositions. Hence, we have argued for a renewed awareness of stories as an analytic tool, and one especially adopted to our moral existence, since stories are designed to effect critical awareness as well as describe a state of affairs.

By calling attention to the narrative context of the standard account, we are not proposing a wholesale rejection of that account or of the theories formed under its inspiration. In fact, the efforts expended on developing contrasting ethical theories (like utilitarianism or formalism) have become part of our legacy, and offer a useful way to introduce one to ethical reasoning. Furthermore, the manner of proceeding which we associate with the standard account embodies concerns which any substantive moral narrative must respect: a high regard for public discourse, the demand that we be able to offer reasons for acting at once cogent and appropriate, and a way to develop critical skills of discrimination and judgment. Finally, any morality depends on a capacity to generate and to articulate moral principles that can set boundaries for proper behavior and guide our conduct.

Our emphasis on narrative need not militate against any of these distinctive concerns. Our difficulty rather lies with the way the standard account attempts to express and to ground these concerns in a manner of accounting which is narrative-free. So we are given the impression that moral principles offer the actual ground for conduct, while in fact they present abstractions whose significance continues to depend on original narrative contexts. Abstractions play useful roles in reasoning, but a continual failure to identify them as abstractions becomes systematically misleading: a concern for rationality thereby degenerates into a form of rationalism.

Our criticism of the standard account has focused on the anomalies which result from that rationalism. We have tried to show how the hegemony of the standard account in ethics has in fact ignored or distorted significant aspects of moral experience. We do not wish to gainsay the importance of rationality for ethics; only to expose a pretentious form of rationalism. Though the point can be made in different ways, it is no accident that the stories which form the lives of Jews and Christians make them peculiarly sensitive to any account which demands that human existence fit a rational framework. The legitimate human concern for rationality is framed by a range of powers of quite another order. It is this larger contingent context which narrative is designed to order in the only manner available to us.

In this way, we offer a substantive explication of narrative as a constructive alternative to the standard account. Our penchant has been to rely upon the standard account as though it were the only lifeboat in a sea of subjective reactions and reductive explanations. To question it would be tantamount to exposing the leaks in the only bark remaining to us. In harkening to the narrative context for action, we are trying to direct attention to an alternative boat available to us. This one cannot provide the security promised by the other, but in return it contains instructions designed to equip us with the skills required to negotiate the dangers of the open sea.

3. Stories and Reasons for Acting

Ethics deals explicitly with reasons for acting. The trick lies in turning reasons into a form proper to acting. The normal form for reasoning requires propositions to be linked so as to display how the conclusion follows quite naturally. The very skills which allow us to form statements lead us to draw other statements from them as conclusions. The same Aristotle who perfected this art, however, also reminded us that practical syllogisms must conclude in an action rather than another proposition.[23] As syllogisms, they will display the form proper to reasoning, yet they must do so in a way that issues in action.

This difference reflects the fact that practical wisdom cannot claim to be a science, since it must deal with particular courses of action (rather than recurrent patterns); nor can it call itself an art, since "action and making are different kinds of thing." The alternative Aristotle settles for is "a true and reasoned . . . capacity to act with regard to the things that are good or bad for man" (*N. Ethics,* 1140b5). We have suggested that stories in fact help us all to develop that capacity as a reasoned capacity. This section will focus on the narrative form as a form of rationality; the following section will show how the act of discriminating among stories develops skills for judging truly what is "good or bad for man." Using Aristotle's discriminations as a point of reference is meant to indicate that our thesis could be regarded as a development of his; in fact, we would be pleased to find it judged to be so.

(Our argument put in traditional terms is that the moral life must be grounded in the "nature" of man. However, that "nature" is not "rationality" itself, but the necessity of having a narrative to give our life coherence. The truthfulness of our moral life cannot be secured by claims of "rationality" in itself but rather by the narrative that forms our need to recognize the many claims on our lives without trying to subject them to a false unity of coherence.)

3.1 Narrative Form as Rational Discourse

There are many kinds of stories, and little agreement on how to separate them into kinds. We distinguish short stories from novels, while acknowledging the short novel as well. We recognize that some stories offer with a particular lucidity patterns or plots which recur in countless other stories. We call these more archetypal stories "myths," and often use them as a shorthand for referring to a typical tangle or dilemma which persons find themselves facing, whether in a story or in real life. That feature common to all stories which gives them their peculiar aptitude for illuminating real-life situations is their narrative structure.

Experts will want to anatomize narrative as well, of course, but for our purposes let it be the connected description of action and of suffering which moves to a point. The point need not be detachable from the narrative itself; in fact, we think a story better that does not issue in a determinate *moral*. The "point" we call attention to here has to do with that form of connectedness which characterizes a novel. It is not the mere material connection of happenings to one individual, but the connected unfolding that we call *plot*. Difficult as this is to characterize—independently of displaying it in a good story!—we can nonetheless identify it as a connection among elements (actions, events, situations) which is neither one of logical consequence nor one of mere sequence. The connection seems rather designed to move our understanding of a situation forward by developing or unfolding it. We have described this movement as gathering to a point. Like implication, it seeks to make explicit what would otherwise remain implicit; unlike implication, the rules of development are not those of logic but stem from some more mysterious source.

The rules of development are not logical rules because narrative connects contingent events. The intelligibility which plot affords is not a necessary one, because the events connected do not exhibit recurrent patterns. Narrative is not required to be explanatory, then, in the sense in which a scientific theory must show necessary connections among occurrences. What we demand of a narrative is that it display how occurrences are actions. Intentional behavior is purposeful but not necessary. We are not possessed of the theoretical capacities to predict what will happen on the basis of what has occurred. Thus a narrative moves us on to answer the question that dogs us: what happened next? It cannot answer that question by arbitrary statement, for our inquiring minds are already involved in the process. Yet the question is a genuine one precisely because we lack the capacity for sure prediction.

It is the intentional nature of human action which evokes a narrative account. We act for an end, yet our actions affect a field of forces in ways that may be characteristic yet remain unpredictable. So we can ask, What would follow from our hiring Jones?, as though certain events might be deduced from his coming on board. Yet we also know that whatever follows will not do so deductively, but rather as a plot unfolds. Nevertheless, we are right in inquiring into what might *follow from* our hiring him, since we must act responsibly. By structuring a plausible response to the question, And what happened next?, narrative offers just the intelligibility we need for acting properly.

3.2 What the Narrative Unfolds

But what makes a narrative plausible? The field of a story is actions (either deeds or dreams) or their opposite, sufferings. In either case, what action or passion is seen to unfold is something we call "character." *Character*, of course, is not a theoretical notion, but merely the name we give to the cumulative source of human actions. Stories themselves attempt to probe that source and discover its inner structure by trying to display how human actions and passions connect with one another to develop a character. As we follow the story, we gain some insight into recurrent connecting patterns, and also some ability to assess them. We learn to recognize different configurations and to rank some characters better than others.

Gradually, then, the characters (or ways of unifying actions) that we can recognize offer patterns for predicting recurring ways of acting. Expectations are set up, and the way an individual or others deal with those expectations shows us some of the capacities of the human spirit. In this way, character can assume the role of an analytic tool even though it is not itself an explanatory notion. Character is neither explanatory in origin nor in use, for it cannot be formulated prior to nor independently of the narrative which develops it. Yet it can play an illuminating or analytic role by calling attention to what is going on in a narrative as the plot unfolds: a character is being developed. Moreover, this character, as it develops, serves as a relative baseline for further developing itself or other characters, as we measure subsequent actions and responses against those anticipated by the character already developed. In this way, character plays an analytic role by offering a baseline for further development. That the baseline itself will shift represents one more way of distinguishing narrative development from logical implication.

We may consider the set of expectations associated with a developing character as a "language," a systematic set of connections between actions which offers a setting or syntax for subsequent responses. Since character cannot be presented independently of the story or stories that develop it, however, the connection between a syntactical system and use, or the way in which a language embodies a form of life, becomes crystal clear. By attending to character, stories will display this fact to us without any need for philosophical reminders.

Similarly, we will see how actions, like expressions, accomplish what they do as part of a traditional repertoire. What a narrative must do is to set out the antecedent actions in such a way as to clarify how the resulting pattern becomes a tradition. In this way, we will see why certain actions prove effective and others fail, much as some expressions succeed in saying what they mean while others cannot. Some forms of story, like the three-generation Victorian novel, are expressly designed to display how a grammar for actions develops, by adopting a deliberately historical (even explicitly generational) structure. Lawrence's *Rainbow,* for example, shows how the shaping habits of speech and personal interaction are altered over three generations in response to industrial development. As he skilfully displays this alteration in grammar over against a traditional syntax, we can grasp something of the capacities latent in us as human beings. In articulating the characters. Lawrence succeeds in making explicit some reaches of the human spirit as yet unexplored.

Stories, then, certainly offer more than entertainment. What they do offer, however, cannot be formulated independently of our appreciating the story, so seeking entertainment is less distracting than looking for a moral. The reason lies with the narrative structure, whose plot cannot be abstracted without banality, yet whose unity does depend on its having a point. Hence it is appropriate to speak of a plot, to call attention to the ordering peculiar to narrative. It is that ordering, that capacity to unfold or develop character, and thus offer insight into the human conditions, which recommends narrative as a form of rationality especially appropriate to ethics.

3.3   How a Narrative Unfolds

If a narrative becomes plausible as it succeeds in displaying a believable character, we may still ask how *that* achievement offers us an intelligibility appropriate to discriminating among courses of action. Using Aristotle's language, how can stories assist in the formation of a practical wisdom? How can stories themselves develop a capacity for judging among alternatives? And further, how does discriminating among stories make that capacity even keener? Since reading stories for more than mere entertainment is usually described as "appreciating" them, some skills for assessing among them are already implied in one's appreciating any single story.

We often find ourselves quite unable, however, to specify the grounds for preferring one story to another. Critics, of course, develop a language for doing this, trying to formulate our normally inchoate criteria. Yet these criteria themselves are notoriously ambiguous. They must be rendered in utterly analogous terms, like 'unity', 'wholeness', 'consistency', 'integrity', etc. So we cannot hope to grasp the criteria without a paradigm instance, yet how present an exemplary instance without telling a story?[24] So criticism can only conceive itself as disciplining our native capacity to appreciate a good story.

A complete account of the way narrative functions, then, would be a narrative recounting how one came to judge certain stories better than others. Since this narrative would have to be autobiographical, we would have a vantage for judgment beyond the intrinsic merit of the narrative itself, in the perceived character of its author. If stories are designed to display how one might create and relate to a world and so offer us a paradigm for adopting a similar posture, this autobiographical story would have to show how a person's current manner of relating himself to the world itself represents a posture towards alternative stances. The narrative will have to recount why—and do so in the fashion proper to narrative—one stance comes after another, preferably by improving upon it.[25]

Augustine's *Confessions* offer just such an account by showing how Augustine's many relationships, all patterned on available stories, were gradually relativized to one overriding and ordering relationship with God revealing himself in Jesus. Augustine's life-story is the story of that process of ordering.

3.4 Augustine's Confessions: *A Narrative Assessment of Life Stories*

Writing ten years after the decisive moment in the garden, Augustine sees that event as culminating a quest shaped by two questions: How to account for evil? How to conceive of God? That quest was also dogged by demands much more immediate than questions, of course. These needs were symbolically ordered in the experience recounted in Book 9, and monitored sense by sense, passion by passion, in Book 10. What interests us here, however, is the step-wise manner in which Augustine relates himself relating to the shaping questions: How explain evil? How conceive divinity?

The pear-tree story allows him to telegraph to the reader how he was able to discriminate one question from the other early on, even though the skills developed to respond to one would help him meet the other. For his own action, reflected upon, allowed him to glimpse an evil deed as wanton or pointless (2.4-10). From the perspective displayed by the *Confessions,* he formulates clearly an intimation which guided his earlier quest: what makes an action evil is not so much a reason as the lack of one. So we would be misled to attribute evil to the creator who orders all things, since ordering and giving reasons belong together.

By separating in this way the query into the source of evil from the attempt to conceive divinity, Augustine took a categorical step. That is, he was learning how to slip from the grip in which Manichean teaching held him, as he came to realize that nothing could properly explain the presence of evil in the world. Nothing, that is, short of a quality of human freedom which allowed us to act for no reason at all. Since explanations offer reasons, and evil turns on the lack of reasons, some form other than a causal explanation must be called for. The only form which can exhibit an action without pretending to explain it is the very one he adopted for the book itself: narrative. So Augustine took his first decisive step towards responding to the shaping questions by eschewing the pretense of explanation in favor of a reflective story.

Categorical discriminations are not usually made all at once, of course. If we are set to turn up an explanation, we will ordinarily keep trying to find a satisfactory one. We cannot give up the enterprise of looking for an explanation unless our very horizon shifts. (It is just such a horizon shift or paradigm change which we identify as a categorical discrimination.) Yet horizons form the stable background for inquiry, so normally we cannot allow them to shift. In Augustine's case, as in many, it only occurred to him to seek elsewhere after repeated attempts at explaining proved fruitless. Furthermore, the specific way in which the Manichean scheme failed to explain the presence of evil also suggested why seeking an explanation was itself a fruitless tack.

To be sure, the Manichean accounts to which Augustine alludes strike us as altogether too crude to qualify as explanations. In fact, it sounds odd to identify his rejection of Manichean teachings with the explicit adoption of a story-form, since it is their schemes which sound to us like "stories." The confusion is understandable enough, of course; it is the very one this essay addresses: stories are fanciful, while explanations are what offer intelligibility. Yet fanciful as they appear to us, the Manichean schemes are explanatory in form. They postulate causes for behavior in the form of diverse combinations of "particles" of light or darkness. The nature of the particles is less relevant, of course, than the explanatory pretense.

What first struck Augustine was the scheme's inability to explain diverse kinds of behavior coherently (5.10, 7.1-6). What he came to realize, however, was that *any* explanatory scheme would in principle undermine a person's ability to repent because it would remove whatever capacity we might have for assuming responsibility for our own actions (6.5, 7.12–13, 8.10). This capacity to assume responsibility would not always suffice to accomplish what we (or at least a part of us) desire (8.8–9); but such a capacity is logically necessary if we are to claim our actions as our own—and so receive praise or blame for them. If our contrary actions could be explained by contrary substances within us, then we would not be able to own them. And if we cannot own our actions, then we have no self to speak of. So the incoherence of the explanations offered led Augustine to see how the very quest for explanation itself failed to cohere with the larger life project belonging to every person.

As the narrative of Augustine's own life project displays, this deliberate shift away from the explanatory modes of the Manichees or the astrologers led to adopting a form which would also help him better to conceive divinity. If evil is senseless, we cannot attribute it to the one who creates with order and reason. If we commit evil deeds, we must be able to own up to them, to confess them, if we want to open ourselves to a change of heart. And the more we examine that self which can act responsibly—in accomplishing deeds or in judging among opinions—the more we come into possession of a language for articulating divinity. It was a language of inwardness, as practiced by the Platonists of his day (7.10). It assumed a scheme of powers of the soul, but made its point by transcendental argument: if we are to make the discriminations we do, we must do so by virtue of an innate light or power (7.17). This way of articulating the power by which we act responsibly, then, becomes the model for expressing divinity. The path which led away from seeking an explanation for evil offers some promise for responding to the second question as well.

Augustine must take one more step, however, lest he forfeit the larger lesson of his struggle with the Manichees, and simply substitute a Platonist explanatory scheme for theirs.[26] They appeal to formal facts by way of transcendental argument. His life, however, was framed by facts of another kind: of rights and wrongs dealt to others (6.15); of an order to which he now aspired to conform, but which he found himself unable to accomplish (8.11). What he misses in the Platonists' book is "the mien of the true love of God. They make no mention of the tears of confession" (7.21). He can read there "of the Word, God . . . but not read in them that 'the Word was made flesh and came to dwell among us' (John 1:14)" (7.9). While they speak persuasively of the conditions for acting and judging aright, they do not tell us how to do what we find ourselves unable to do: to set our hearts aright.

The key to that feat Augustine finds not in the books of the Platonists, but in the gospels. Or better, he finds it in allowing the stories of the gospels to shape his story. The moment of permission, as he records it, is preceded by stories of others allowing the same to happen to them, recounting how they did it and what allowing it to happen did to them. The effect of these stories is to insinuate a shift in grammar tantamount to the shift from explanation to narrative, though quite in line with that earlier shift. Since we think of stories as relating accomplishments, Augustine must use these stories together with his own to show us another way of conceiving them.

It is not a new way, for it consciously imitates the biblical manner of displaying God's great deeds in behalf of his people. Without ceasing to be the story of Israel, the tales of the Bible present the story of God. Similarly, without ceasing to be autobiography, Augustine's *Confessions* offer an account of God's way with him. The language of will and of struggle is replaced by that of the heart: ''As I came to the end of the sentence, it was as though the light of confidence flooded into my heart and all the darkness of doubt was dispelled'' (8.12). Yet the transformation is not a piece of magic; the narrative testifies to that. And his narrative will give final testimony to the transformation of that moment in the measure that it conforms to the life story of the ''Word made flesh.'' So the answer to his shaping questions is finally received rather than formulated, and that reception is displayed in the narrative we have analyzed.

4.   Truthfulness as Veracity and Faithfulness

The second step which Augustine relates is not a categorial one. It no longer has to do with finding the proper form for rendering a life project intelligible. The narrative Augustine tells shows us how he was moved to accept the gospel story by allowing it to shape his own. In more conventional terms, this second step moves beyond philosophical therapy to a judgment of truth. That is why recognizable arguments surround the first step, but not this one. Assent involves more subtle movements than clarification—notably assent of this sort, which is not an assent *to* evidence but an assent *of* faith. Yet we will grasp its peculiar warrants better if we see how it moves along the same lines as the categorial discrimination.

Accepting a story as normative by allowing it to shape one's own story in effect reinforces the categorial preference for story over explanation as a vehicle of understanding. Augustine adumbrates the way one step leads into the other towards the beginning of Book 6:

> From now on I began to prefer the Catholic teaching. The Church demanded that certain things should be believed even though they could not be proved. . . . I thought that the Church was entirely honest in this and far less pretentious than the Manichees, who laughed at people who took things on faith, made rash promises of scientific knowledge, and then put forward a whole system of preposterous inventions which they expected their followers to believe on trust because they could not be proved. (6.5)

The chapter continues in a similar vein, echoing many contemporary critiques of modern rationalist pretensions.

4.1   Criteria for Judging among Stories

The studied preference for story over explanation, then, moves one into a neighborhood more amenable to what thirteenth-century theologians called an "assent of faith," and in doing so, helps us develop a set of criteria for judging among stories. Books 8, 9, and 10 of the *Confessions* record the ways in which this capacity for discriminating among stories is developed. It is less a matter of weighing arguments than of displaying how adopting different stories will lead us to become different sorts of persons. The test of each story is the sort of person it shapes. When examples of diverse types are offered to us for our acceptance, the choices we make display in turn our own grasp of the *humanum*. Aristotle presumed we could not fail to recognize a just man, but also knew he would come in different guises (*N. Ethics* 1097b6–1098b7).

The criteria for judging among stories, then, will most probably not pass an impartial inspection. For the powers of recognition cannot be divorced from one's own capacity to recognize the good for humankind. This observation need not amount to a counsel of despair, however. It is simply a reminder that on matters of judgment we consult more readily with some persons than others, because we recognize them to be in a better position to weigh matters sensibly. Any account of that "position" would have to be autobiographical, of course. But it is not an account we count on; it is simply our recognition of the person's integrity.

Should we want to characterize the story which gives such coherence to a person's life, however, it would doubtless prove helpful to contrast it with alternatives. The task is a difficult one, however, either for oneself or for another. For we cannot always identify the paths we have taken; Augustine continued to be engaged in mapping out the paths he was actually traversing at the very time of composing the *Confessions* (*vide* Book 10). Yet we can certainly formulate a list of working criteria, provided we realize that any such list cannot pretend to completeness nor achieve unambiguous expression.

Any story which we adopt, or allow to adopt us, will have to display:

(1) power to release us from destructure alternatives;
(2) ways of seeing through current distortions;
(3) room to keep us from having to resort to violence;
(4) a sense for the tragic: how meaning transcends power.

It is inaccurate, of course, to list these criteria as features which a story must display. For they envisage rather the effect which stories might be expected to have on those who allow them to shape their lives. The fact that stories are meant to be read, however, forces one to speak of them as relational facts. So we cannot help regarding a story as something which (when well-constructed) will help us develop certain skills of perception and understanding. This perspective corresponds exactly to the primary function of narratives by contrast with explanatory schemes: to relate us to the world, including our plans for modifying it. Those plans have consequences of their own, but their shape as well as their execution depends on the expectations we entertain for planning.

Those expectations become a part of the plans themselves, but they can be articulated independently. And when they are, they take the form of stories, notably of heroes. Thus the process of industrialization becomes the story of tycoons, as the technology we know embodies a myth of man's dominating and transforming the earth. Not that industrial processes are themselves stories, or technological expertise a myth. In fact, we are witnessing today many attempts to turn those processes and that expertise to different ends by yoking them to a different outlook. Stories of these experiments suggest new ways of using some of the skills we have developed, and illustrate the role of narrative in helping us to formulate and to practice new perspectives.[27]

Stories, then, help us, as we hold them, to relate to our world and our destiny: the origins and goals of our lives, as they embody in narrative form specific ways of acting out that relatedness. So in allowing ourselves to adopt and be adopted by a particular story, we are in fact assuming a set of practices which will shape the ways we relate to our world and destiny. Lest this sound too instrumental, we should remind ourselves that the world is not simply waiting to be seen, but that language and institutions train us to regard it in certain ways.[28] The criteria listed above assume this fact; let us consider them in greater detail.

4.2　Testing the Criteria

Stories which (2) offer ways to see through current distortions can also (1) empower us to free ourselves from destructive alternatives. For we can learn how to see a current ideology as a distortion by watching what it can do to people who let it shape their story. The seduction of Manichean doctrine for Augustine and his contemporaries lay precisely in its offering itself as a *story* for humankind—much as current problem-solving techniques will invariably also be packaged as a set of practices leading to personal fulfillment. So Augustine's subsequent discrimination between explanation and story first required an accurate identification of Manichean teaching as explanatory pretense in the guise of a story.

To judge an alternative course to be destructive, of course, requires some experience of its effects on those who practice the skills it embodies. It is the precise role of narrative to offer us a way of experiencing those effects without experimenting with our own lives as well. The verisimilitude of the story, along with its assessable literary structure, will allow us to ascertain whether we can trust it as a vehicle of insight, or whether we are being misled. In the absence of narratives, recommendations for adopting a set of practices can only present themselves as a form of propaganda, and be judged accordingly.[29] Only narrative can allow us to take the measure of a scheme for human improvement, granting that we possess the usual skills for discriminating among narratives as well.

The last two criteria also go together: (3) providing room to keep us from having to resort to violence, and (4) offering a sense for the tragic: how meaning transcends power. We can watch these criteria operate if we contrast the story characteristic to Christians and Jews with one of the prevailing presumptions of contemporary culture: that we can count on technique to offer eventual relief from the human condition. This conviction is reflected in the penchant of consequential ethical theories not only to equate doing one's duty with the greatest good for all, but also to presume that meeting our obligations will provide the satisfaction we seek. Surely current medical practice is confirmed by the conviction that harnessing more human energies into preventing and curing disease will increasingly free our lives from tragic dilemmas.[30] Indeed, science as a moral enterprise has provided what Ernest Becker has called an anthropodicy, as it holds out the possibility that our increased knowledge serves human progress toward the creation of a new human ideal, namely, to create a mankind free of suffering.[31]

But this particular ethos has belied the fact that medicine, at least as characterized by its moral commitment to the individual patient, is a tragic profession. For to attend to one in distress often means many others cannot be helped. Or to save a child born retarded may well destroy the child's family and cause unnecessary burdens on society. But the doctor is pledged to care for each patient because medicine does not aim at some ideal moral good, but to care for the needs of the patient whom the doctor finds before him. Because we do not know how to regard medicine as a tragic profession, we tend of course to confuse caring with curing. The story which accompanies technology—of setting nature aright—results in the clinical anomalies to which we are subjecting others and ourselves in order to avoid the limits of our existence.[32]

The practice of medicine under the conditions of finitude offers an intense paradigm of the moral life. For the moral task is to learn to continue to do the right, to care for this immediate patient, even when we have no assurance that it will be the successful thing to do. To live morally, in other words, we need a substantive story that will sustain moral activity in a finite and limited world. Classically, the name we give such stories is tragedy. When a culture loses touch with the tragic, as ours clearly has done, we must redescribe our failures in acceptable terms. Yet to do so *ipso facto* traps us in self-deceiving accounts of what we have done.[33] Thus our stories quickly acquire the characteristics of a policy, especially as they are reinforced by our need to find self-justifying reasons for our new-found necessities.

This tactic becomes especially troublesome as the policy itself assumes the form of a central story that gives our individual and collective lives coherence. This story then becomes indispensable to us, as it provides us with a place to be. Phrases like "current medical practice," "standard hospital policy," or even "professional ethics," embody exemplary stories which guide the way we use the means at hand to care for patients. Since we fail to regard them as stories, however, but must see them as a set of principles, the establishment must set itself to secure them against competing views. If the disadvantaged regard this as a form of institutional violence, they are certainly correct.

Such violence need not take the form of physical coercion, of course. But we can detect it in re-descriptions which countenance coercion. So, for example, an abortion at times may be a morally necessary, but sorrowful, occurrence. But our desire for righteousness quickly invites us to turn what is morally unavoidable into a self-deceiving policy, e.g., the fetus, after all, is just another piece of flesh. It takes no mean skill, certainly, to know how to hold onto a description that acknowledges significant life, while remaining open to judging that it may have to be destroyed. Yet medical practice and human integrity cannot settle for less. Situations like these suggest, however, that we do not lie because we are evil, but because we wish to be good or preserve what good we already embody.[34]

We do not wish to claim that the stories with which Christians and Jews identify are the only stories that offer skills for truthfulness in the moral life. We only want to identify them as ways to countenance a posture of locating and doing the good which must be done, even if it does not lead to human progress. Rather than encourage us to assume that the moral life can be freed from the tragedies that come from living in a limited and sinful world, these stories demand that we be faithful to God as we believe he has been faithful to us through his covenant with Israel and (for Christians) in the cross of Christ.[35]

4.3   A Canonical Story

Religious faith, on this account, comes to accepting a certain set of stories as canonical. We come to regard them not only as meeting the criteria sketched above, along with others we may develop, but find them offering ways of clarifying and expanding our sense of the criteria themselves. In short, we discover our human self more effectively through these stories, and so use them in judging the adequacy of alternative schemes for humankind.

In this formal sense, one is tempted to wonder whether everyone does not accept a set of stories as canonical. To identify those stories would be to discover the shape one's basic convictions take. To be unable to do so would either mark a factual incapacity or an utterly fragmented self. Current discussion of "polytheism" leads one to ask whether indiscriminate pluralism represents a real psychic possibility for a contemporary person.[36] In our terms, arguing against the need for a canonical story amounts to questioning "why be good?" Just as we do not require ethics to answer that question, so we need not demand a perspicuously canonical story. But we can point to the endemic tendency of men and women to allow certain stories to assume that role, just as ethicists remind us of the assessments we do in fact count on to live our lives.

2. Obligation and Virtue Once More

> It does seem to me that moral philosophy must do more than hint at an ethics of virtue in a footnote—or in an article or chapter. It must fully explore the possibility of a satisfactory ethics of virtue as an alternative or supplement to one of obligation and moral goodness, not only to explain what the people we admire in biography and literature live by, but to see what there is in our "new morality" and how we ourselves should or at least may live.
>
> William K. Frankena[1]

1. The Ethics of Virtue as a Problem

This quotation sets the intention of this essay in which I intend to explore why and how the concept of virtue might be more than a footnote. Frankena's work provides ready access to this endeavor. He has been one of the few philosophers from the side of obligation to try to account for the significance of the concept of virtue for the moral life. However, I will argue that Frankena, because of his insistence on the primacy of the ethics of obligation, has failed to provide a satisfactory account of the interdependent relationship of virtue and obligation.[2]

Frankena in his characteristic fashion has defined the problem that is central for this essay. He has tried to come to terms with Prichard's observation that when one turns from the "vivid accounts of human life and action" found in Shakespeare to moral philosophy, the latter seems remote and abstract from the facts of life. With Prichard, Frankena[3] thinks the explanation for this is due to moral philosophy's correct concentration on the theory of obligation as the determination of morality even though "many *admirable* people live by something other than a sense of moral obligation or an ideal of moral goodness." Through my criticism of Frankena I will try to provide an account of morality that does justice both to the language of obligation and to the fact that such language alone fails to constitute how we learn to live morally.

In concentrating on this problem my underlying interest is also shared by Frankena. For while Frankena continues to criticize attempts to construct an ethics of virtue, he nonetheless returns to it time and time again, suspecting that it has an importance that we have not yet learned how rightly to appreciate. It is my thesis that its importance lies exactly in the attempt to restore the

> integration and cooperation between man's beliefs about the world in which he lives (Ises) and his beliefs about the values and purposes that should direct his conduct (Oughts) (as this) is the deepest problem of modern life. (And) It is the problem of any philosophy that is not isolated from that life.[4]

This kind of integration can come only when we cease thinking of moral conduct primarily as an affair of obligation and instead see that most of what we do is done in order to maintain our sense of who we are. Put starkly, integrity, not obligation, is the hallmark of the moral life.[5]

1.1　The Argument in Summary

My analysis of Frankena's position involves three main arguments: A. I argue that all the desires and interests which form the basis of the conflicts which morality is designed to arbitrate cannot be understood apart from a conception of the moral agent and what sort of life is best suited for him. In this connection I will claim that Frankena has an insufficient moral psychology and as a result fails to see that our desires and interests are subject to, formed by, and yet direct our practical reason. B. I will maintain that we cannot understand the motivational force of "ought judgments" apart from a conception of formed human character to which these judgments appeal. We can only use ought judgments because we presuppose certain characteristics in others and ourselves that make our "oughts" intelligible. C. I argue that the *descriptions* (or notions) of actions which provide the material content of our ought statements always contain assumptions and stipulations of the agent's intentions. It is only because we take such intentions for granted that we think our moral notions can be isolated as an ethics of obligation devoid of any reference to the kind of agent we are.

These three arguments are interrelated. I assume that Frankena will agree or partially agree with the arguments, but the issue is their systematic implications for how one conceives of "morality." I hope to show that if these arguments are correct, then Frankena's claim for the independence of the "institution of morality" must be qualified insofar as this claim is dependent on the existence or the primacy of "an ethics of obligation."

1.2　The Importance of Virtue-Obligation for Religion-Morality

Toward the end of this essay I suggest how and why the question of the relation of virtue and obligation has important implications for our under-

standing the relation between religion and morality. Just as it has been a
mistake to cast the relation between virtue and obligation in terms of priority
and in some cases dependence, the same mistake has also dominated discussions of the relation of religion and morality. Morality is no more "dependent" on religion than virtue is "dependent" on obligation. The relation is
not one of priority, either conceptually, logically or causally, but rather of
how each contributes to the formation of the moral self.

When ethics is identified primarily as a matter of obligation divorced from
an ethics of virtue, one fails to see how religious convictions embody and
order the moral life. For then religious beliefs, like virtues, are relegated to
the motivational or subjective side of the moral life where they can have no
possible bearing on the way the moral life is conceived or lived. Hence the
contemporary emphasis on the ethics of obligation has misplaced the relation
of religious convictions to the moral life. And that relation represents but one
aspect of the necessary integration of our beliefs and conduct, our virtues and
our duties.

1.3   Virtue-Obligation as a Problem for Theological Ethics

The question of the relation between the language of obligation and virtue
then is clearly more than a philosophical problem. As Carney[6] has recently
shown, the relation bears directly on theological ethics. Hence my interest in
Frankena's understanding of the relation of virtue to obligation: the problems
with which he is dealing are also problems with which theological ethicists
must deal in their effort to explicate the grammar of religious convictions.

This is particularly true for my own work as I have concentrated almost
entirely on trying to develop an ethics of character.[7] I have done this partly
because I have found the language of obligation ill-suited to expressing issues
of theological ethics as *the* language of morality. (My criticism of the concentration on decision and acts as the hallmark of the moral life has been but a
corollary of my deeper dissatisfaction with the language of obligation as the
dominant form of construing the moral life.) By trying to come to terms with
Frankena's understanding of the ethics of obligation, I will also be trying to
spell out more adequately how my own position can account for the language
of obligation.

2.   The "Pure" Theory of Virtue

I am puzzled that Frankena[8] thinks it important to construct a "pure"
theory of virtue. As an analytic exercise or as a "type," such a procedure

cannot be objected to. But there are indications that Frankena's construction of a "pure" theory of virtue is more than an analytical type. For if a pure theory of virtue, by which Frankena means a theory not dependent on any explicit or implicit account of obligation, can be shown deficient in a significant way, then it would seem to establish the necessity or priority of a "pure" ethics of obligation. (By a "pure" theory of obligation I do not mean to suggest that such a theory would necessarily exclude all virtues but rather that virtues, regardless of their character, would be obligation-derived and dependent. Frankena has always maintained that "principles without virtues are impotent," but such virtues are required by duties that are determined free of all considerations of virtue.)

Yet I have no stake in defending anything like what Frankena understands as a "pure" theory of virtue. Indeed such a theory has all the marks of a red herring. Rather I will try to show—and, as I think, aspects of Frankena's own theory of obligation illustrate—that the languages of virtue and obligation are interdependently related. At this point, however, we can see that Frankena's further attempts to characterize and contrast virtue and obligation only reveal the difficulty of trying to separate a "pure" theory of virtue from the language of obligation, and vice versa.

2.1 Two Difficulties with the Contrast between Obligation and Virtue

Frankena tries to contrast the ethics of virtue and obligation in at least two different ways. Thus he suggests that, "deontic terms and judgments are more like legal ones than aretaic terms and judgments are; ... that aretaic judgments can be made of both actions and persons, as well as motives and intentions, whereas deontic judgments are more properly made of actions than of persons, motives, or intentions; and that a reference to motives and intentions is involved in aretaic judgments in a way in which it is not in deontic ones."[9] Yet to make the contrast between an ethics of virtue and obligation in this manner is misleading, for it assumes an unwarranted separation of intention from actions. Frankena is right that an ethics of virtue tends to stress the importance of the agent's perspective (which is not the same as the agent's judgment), but as I will try to show, it need not do this at the expense of public criteria and description of action.[10] Nor is the language of obligation, even when limited to judgments about discrete actions, devoid of assumptions about the intentions of the agent performing the act.

In another context[11] Frankena employs Mandelbaum's distinction between direct and removed moral judgments as a way of specifying the relation between virtue and obligation. "Direct moral judgments are those in which a person as agent judges what actions or kinds of actions it is right, good, or virtuous for him to do in the situations that face him. Removed moral judgments are those in which a person is judging as a spectator, judging the actions done by others, the character of others, his past actions, or his own character.'' Frankena observes that an ethics of virtue must not only guide a spectator in making removed judgments, but must also guide the agent in direct judgments of what to do. An ethics of virtue might limit itself only to removed moral judgments, such as looking back on one's life, but then it would not be offering us anything to live by. ''For such guidance we will still have to look to an ethics of duty—or simply follow our desires, passions and interests, unaided and unmodified by any ideal or principle, moral or non-moral.''[12]

Frankena, however, later qualifies this judgment.[13] Here he suggests there are at least two ways a ''pure'' ethics of virtue might serve as a ''guide for life'': (1) it can tell us to become loving and then do what love (using its head) tells us to do; or (2) it can simply suggest with Aristotle that we should do what the loving man would do, assuming that such a man could be located and that we would know what he would do. (Though I do not wish to argue historically, Frankena's appeals to Aristotle tend to be misleading. Aristotle's emphasis on virtue cannot be divorced from his analysis of human activity.)[14]

A third possibility, not considered by Frankena, is that virtue can guide our behavior inasmuch as virtues form the self. Frankena seems to assume that any ''guide to life'' must primarily involve a decision procedure for particular actions. But morally our lives are not made up just of discrete decisions or choices, but include the marks of our underlying character. The virtues are therefore ''a guide to life'' inasmuch as our life is more than the responses we make to particular situations. Our choices are never simply given, but rather are what they are because we are what we are.

These difficulties indicate that Frankena has simply not provided a sufficient account of how virtue and obligation may be related. I suspect part of his difficuty involves his assumption that ethics is somehow committed to articulating a ''basic guide to life.''[15] For Frankena, therefore, an ethics of virtue appears to be an attempt to substitute judgments of persons, traits or dispositions for judgments of actions as the ''basic guide to life.'' But there is no immediately apparent reason why an ethics of virtue should involve such a commitment; even so, Frankena is indeed correct that an ethics of virtue does not separate the characterization of an act from the reason the agent performed it. The demand for such a separation, and the resulting contrast between virtue and obligation, results not from the nature of the ethics of virtue, but from Frankena's (and Prichard's) concern to secure the independence of morality in the form of the language of obligation; or perhaps more accurately put, from a concern to distinguish morality from all particular moral systems.[16]

2.2   *Virtue and Moral Psychology*

Although Frankena's argument makes it difficult to display the relation between virtue and obligation in terms of direct and removed moral judgments, more needs to be said about this than is involved in his change of mind. His discussion of this distinction implies an unwarranted separation between duty and our desires, passions and interests. It is the primary concern of an ethics of virtue to form our interests in a manner that we will do our duty; but more fundamentally, that we will be able to see what duties we have exactly because we are the kind of person we are.

It is, therefore, misleading to say, as Frankena does, that an ethics of virtue is somehow committed to the position: "Be a bundle of love and then do what you please."[17] A more complete ethic of virtue assumes that the man of virtue can be counted on exactly because his desires, passions, and interests have been formed through the practical intelligence. The sense of how virtues determine and guide moral behavior is transformed as soon as it is seen that virtues are not simply emotions, but skills of perception, articulation and action.

I suspect Frankena has failed to see this because he has never been interested in issues of moral psychology. One will search in vain in his work to find an extended analysis of such terms as motive, disposition, feeling or character. He seems content with Prichard's claim that virtues are "dispositions or tendencies to feel and act from intrinsically good desires arising from intrinsically good emotions," but such desires, passions or interests cannot be at the control of our will.[18] Therefore, the ethics of virtue cannot give an intelligible account of how moral language is directive as we cannot be obliged to act from a certain motive since that is not under our control at all.[19]

Though I am not sure Frankena accepts every aspect of Prichard's position, he does seem to presuppose a moral psychology much like this.[20] But surely this fails to note the important difference between dispositions and feelings. The former, as Aristotle and Thomas make clear, are habitual skills of behavior that are under the control of the agent exactly because they have been formed through the practical intelligence. Put differently, Frankena assumes far too easily that the distinction between being and doing is immediately clear. With a more adequate philosophical psychology we see that it is not easy to separate the description of what we do from why we do it as an agent.

For an agent is not related to his action as a cause to an effect, but rather as an agent whose own description continues to determine what he has done. The "effect" (act) is not therefore separable from the agent's intentions any more than the agent's intentions are separable from the "effect." Our intentions and motives, which are the articulations of our interests and desires, are not just subjective "wants," but rather are open to public disclosure and scrutiny. The limits of such disclosure and scrutiny, or better the limits of the rational portrayal of our desires, are but the limits of our language.

For the purposes of this essay, there is no need to distinguish intentions from motives. We can simply treat motives as but one form of intentionality.[21] It is important to observe, however, that the distinction between intentions and motives is not equivalent to the public reasons for my action and my more narrowly biographical or "private" reasons. Intentions are involved more intimately than motives in the description of the action qua description, but this does not mean that our motives are less morally relevant for behavior than our intentions.

As Aquinas insists, for an act to be good "it is not enough to be good in one point only; it must be good in every respect. If therefore the will be good both from its proper object and from its end, it follows that the external action is good. But if the will be good from its intention of the end, this is not enough to make the external action good; and if the will be evil either by reason of its intention or the end, or by reason of the act willed, it follows that the external action is evil."[22] An act must be done in a manner that the doing of it makes the agent good, i.e., from right reason. Our motives are morally significant just to the extent that what we do is not only good, but that we do it as good persons—as people of virtue.

2.3 Virtue, Obligation and the Good Life

Frankena, however, is surely right that an ethics of virtue tends to "make the virtue of an action rest on the virtue of the motive or disposition behind it."[23] Thus only an aretaic agent-ethic, in contrast to aretaic situational ethics or aretaic ethics of principle, is a genuine alternative to an ethics of obligation. The other two forms of virtue ethics are still fundamentally ethics of "doing," whereas an ethics of virtue is concerned with "being."[24] Therefore, an ethics of virtue is committed to the claim that "aretaic judgments about agents and/or their motives or traits are prior to aretaic judgments about actions."[25]

The ethics of virtue may well be related to any conception of the good life, but Prichard's claim that "virtue is no basis for morality" serves merely to call attention to the mistake that makes the morally right dependent on a conception of the non-moral good.[26] Virtues involve dispositions that are actuated, not by duty or a sense of duty, but by some good motive such as generosity or sympathy.[27] Frankena's formulation of a "pure" ethics of virtue is itself an attempt to free "morality" from dependency on "subjective" human emotions or concerns.

In relation to the good life, Frankena[28] maintains "that our lives will be better if we take them or live them in certain ways or frames of mind rather than others—if they have certain 'subjective forms' or 'styles,' to use Whitehead's words. In other words, the *how* of our lives matters to their goodness as well as the *what*. This seems to me to be profoundly true, as long as it is not suggested that the *what* does not matter at all or very much, or that all we need attend to educationally or otherwise is the *how* and the rest will take care of itself." Frankena is therefore more than prepared to argue that a number of attitudes or frames of mind are important for the good life, e.g., objectivity, clear-headedness, discipline, authenticity, honesty, courage, fidelity and even love. However, besides these "frames" our lives must have a design or pattern, or perhaps in more traditional language, character.

2.4 The Alleged Insufficiency of the "Pure" Theory of Virtue

Even though, as we have seen, Frankena qualifies his earlier claim that "virtues without principles are blind,"[29] he still feels that an ethics of virtue involves a fundamental difficulty. For in spite of Anscombe's argument that the "fact of obligation" is a hand-me-down from a discarded divine command theory of ethics, Frankena continues to think, along with Kant and Prichard, that there is "the fact of obligation" and therefore no pure ethics of virtue can be satisfactory.[30]

I have no wish to argue a thesis as radical as Anscombe's or to defend Frankena's sense of a "pure" theory of virtue and obligation because of his concern to establish the "objectivity" of an ethics of obligation.

It may be that Frankena finds Kant and Prichard's claim about "the fact of obligation" accords best with his "own moral consciousness and experience," but I hope to show that if Frankena would look once again at his experience that he would find the "fact of obligation" is more complex than Kant and Prichard's theory would imply. It can easily be shown, when we are not blinded by a theory of obligation, that most of our ought judgments presuppose certain characteristics in those to whom we expect an ought judgment to appeal.

For example, think of all we presuppose in a beginning tennis player when we say, "You ought always to watch the ball into the racket," or "Do not yell at your opponent during play!" Notice that the difference between the grammar of an ought judgment and a command is precisely that "ought" depends on an assumption that the agent has certain characteristics that will secure his obedience. A command, on the other hand, is given in circumstances where regardless of the agent's characteristics one can force him to obey even if he chooses not to do so.

One of the most important conditions for the intelligibility of our ought judgments is that we have certain beliefs about our audience. These beliefs may involve institutional or dispositional expectations. What we have to believe about our audience in order for our moral ought judgments to be made involves more than just a belief in the "fact of obligation" that is putatively grounded in reason. However, in order to sustain this argument we must look more carefully at Frankena's account of the ethics of obligation.

3. The Ethics of Obligation

An ethics of obligation draws its basic force from our experience that we have an obligation to do X even though we may not want or desire to do X. Thus we find nothing logically or morally odd in someone suggesting that we ought to do X even though we do not personally want to do X. This provides the experiential backdrop for Prichard's claim that "the 'fact and the sense of obligation' is and must remain the central fact of both moral experience and moral philosophy, not virtue." Thus Prichard argues that, " 'in the end our obligations are seen to be coextensive with the whole of our life,' though 'even the best men (e.g., those we read about in Shakespeare) are blind to many of their obligations.' "[31]

Correlative of this claim is the assumption that the rightness or wrongness of an act has nothing to do with the question of intention. "There is, and can be, no question of whether I ought to pay my debts from a particular motive. No doubt . . . if we pay our bills we shall pay them with a motive, but in considering whether we ought to pay them we inevitably think of the act in abstraction from the motive."[32] Thus to ask what to do is only to ask what action to do, not what motive to act from.

I find this claim to be significantly wrong. It both distorts how our moral notions work and sunders our intentions from our actions. The moral notions we inherit and learn to use are what they are because of the wants and interests that call them forth. These interests include the kind of agent we ought to be in the doing or not doing of the behavior envisaged by the notion. It is true that we ought not to murder regardless of the motives we have, but we must also observe that for the proper use of the notion "murder" we presuppose certain kinds of intention that the agent must have if we are to use the term at all. Thus, "A proper analysis of a human act must involve reference to intentionality; without it we cannot give a proper description of what we are doing."[33]

This sense of intentionality does not just refer to the subjective conditions of the agent when he performed the act, but is built into how the notion is used to describe the act, whether by the agent himself or by an observer. To say we ought to do or ought not to do something is at the same time to say (contrary to Prichard) that we can have or not have certain kinds of dispositions. Our dispositions and way of being are crucial to make the "ought" work at all, for our "desires" cannot be separated from the description of the act.

Virtues are not feelings or emotions separated from our reasons for action, but rather virtues are the trained skills of the person enabling him to act one way rather than another. The notions that form my dispositions to act one way rather than another are not different from the notions that an observer would use to judge what I ought or ought not to have done.

> What I am arguing for, in effect, is a close connection—a qualified identity— between *explanations* of human action and *reasons* for acting. . . . To explain a want is to make it intelligible. Similarly, the rationality of a man's wants depends upon the possibility of giving reasons for wanting what he wants. To want simply a saucer of mud is irrational, because some further reason is needed for wanting it. To want a saucer of mud because one wants to enjoy its rich river-smell is rational. No further reason is needed for wanting to enjoy the rich river-smell, for to characterize what is wanted as 'to enjoy the rich river-smell' is itself to give an acceptable reason for wanting it, and therefore, this want is rational. . . . The important point, however, is that the characterizations of an action which explain it are *normally* the characterizations that constitute the agent's reasons for performing it.[34]

It may be objected that even if this account of the relationship between our actions and our explanations of our actions is correct I still have failed to make my case. For I have claimed that we must make reference to motives and intentions to indicate what sense it makes to call an act right or wrong at all. However, all I have shown is that one must make references to the agent's intention to explain why the agent acted as he did. This is quite different from a moral justification of the action itself. However, this objection overlooks how notions we use in our justifications already presuppose the intentionality of the agent. We finally cannot separate how we explain our actions from how we morally justify them—unless we are intent on forgetting the actual grammar of our moral notions.

3.1 Justifying and Motivating Reasons

My argument does not challenge the externalist's claim that there is an important distinction between subjective and objective obligation. It may be, as Frankena makes clear, that *assenting* to an obligation may logically entail the existence of a motivation to act accordingly, but this does not mean "that having objectively a certain moral obligation logically entails having some motivation for fulfilling it, that justifying a judgment of objective moral obligation logically implies establishing or producing a motivation buttress, and that it is logically impossible that there should be a state of apprehending a moral obligation of one's own which is not accompanied by such a buttress.''[35]

Moreover, Frankena rightly criticizes the intrinsicalist for failing adequately to distinguish between justifying and motivating reasons. Thus "When A asks, 'Why should I give Smith a ride?' B may give answers of two different kinds. He may say, 'Because you promised to,' or he may say, 'Because, if you do, he will remember you in his will.' In the first case he offers a justification of the action, in the second a motive for doing it. . . . Thus a motive is one kind of reason for action, but not all reasons for action are motives. Perhaps we should distinguish between reasons for acting and reasons for regarding an action as right or justified.''[36]

Frankena does not use this distinction to defend the Kantian view that only when men are motivated wholly by a sense of duty are their actions good. On such a view, any "motivation" other than a sense of duty is "pathological" as it encourages us to act from less than a moral will. For Frankena, however, a "more reasonable view is that a man and his actions are morally good if it is at least true that, whatever his actual motives in acting are, his sense of duty or desire to do the right is so strong in him that it may keep him trying to do his duty anyway.''[37]

While the distinction between justifying and motivating reasons is important, I do not wish to make the distinction in the same manner as Frankena. This is a theory-dependent distinction, since what one understands to be an adequate justifying reason is correlative to what one takes to be the nature of moral justification. Morally justified reasons are, for Frankena, only those that one can defend independently of one's particular interests or wants (one's motives). I think, however, that this can be shown to be misleading even with respect to Frankena's own account of reasons that obligate.

3.2   Obligation and Reason-Giving

According to Frankena, as well as most contemporary ethicists, it is the very genius of morality to appeal to reason, that is, to claim that what one morally should do can be justified. Therefore, "most writers are agreed that the moral approach to questions about action involves being objective, impartial, fact-facing, willing to see one's maxims acted on by everyone even when this is to one's own disadvantage.''[38]

The importance of reason-giving for the moral life shows exactly why the ethics of obligation has played such a prominent role in contemporary ethical reflection. The ethics of obligation places a demand on the agent to give intersubjective reasons that will locate his conduct in a community of discourse wider than his own personal wants. The need to distinguish reasons from "motivation," where the latter is identified with virtues and feeling, is drawn from the need to establish the independence of moral reason from our subjective wishes and wants.

Frankena is certainly aware that when we use ethical and value language we are usually using terms in a manner that shows we have some emotional attitude in relation to them. "But it seems obvious to me that in our actual ethical and value judgments, when we are not frightened out of our normative wits by the relativists, subjectivists, and sceptics, we are not merely exclaiming, commanding, expressing emotion, evoking a response, or committing ourselves; rather, we are claiming some kind of status, justification or validity for our attitudes or judgments."[39] Thus normative judgments cannot be reduced to emotional expressions or even commitments, for by so doing it would bar us from "something it would be less than human not to want to do, namely to claim for ourselves at least a modicum of impersonal rationality and validity."[40]

3.3   Virtue and Reason-Giving

Yet an ethics of virtue demands no less than an ethics of obligation that appropriate reasons be given in explanation and justification for our moral behavior. Virtues are not private emotions that are in principle non-public; virtues are precisely the dispositions formed by reasons that make our explanations for our actions *our* explanations. The difference between an ethics of virtue and obligation is not the activity of reason-giving, but rather the kinds of reasons that are seen to count as "rational."

A stress on obligation tends to characterize "reasons" as those that only an impartial spectator would give to explain an agent's discrete acts. My position, however, is that the notions through which we form our behavior and shape the self determine certain patterns of rational explanation that include the agent's point of view. The defense against a hard relativism cannot lie in the presumption that there is a "reason" that can assure complete objectivity, for our rationality is always context-dependent on the kind of men we are or ought to be. In the words of Aiken that Frankena[41] quotes approvingly, "All that needs defending is the thesis that moral reasoning has its own properties which, while certainly not written into the starry heavens above, are at least constant and extensive enough to enable the members of a given civilization to distinguish a good reason from a bad one." But what allows members to make these distinctions is, at least in part, the kind of persons they have become through the moral traditions of their civilization.

Stuart Hampshire has argued a similar position in his extremely interesting essay, "Morality and Pessimism." Hampshire's primary concern here is to attack utilitarianism, but he also takes aim at a view of moral reason that utilitarians share with much contemporary moral philosophy. This view assumes that moral reason ideally should be able to establish that certain things should be done or forbidden by the "comparatively detached arguments of the sophisticated moralist, who discounts his intuitive responses as being prejudices inherited from an uncritical past."[42] Injunctions concerning duties in time of war, conditions under which truth may be told or concealed, and duties of friendship are hopefully inferable from a "few basic principles, corresponding to the axioms of a theory."[43]

Hampshire argues that to show that certain vices are indeed vices necessarily takes "one back to the criteria for the assessment of persons as persons, and therefore to the whole way of life that one aspires to as the best way of life."[44] The connection between injunctions and obligations that make up our lives is not that forged by impartial reason, but is rather "found in the coherence of a single way of life, distinguished by the characteristic virtues and vices recognized within it."[45]

Hampshire is not suggesting that we simply choose our way of life and then declare arbitrarily that only that which falls within that way of life can be rational. Reason is significant insofar as it is inherently governed by the lessons and experience of men. Similarly the unity and consistency of a "way of life" cannot be derived from an abstractly posited "rationality," but rather is learned "from observation, direct experience, and from psychology and history."[46] Moral prohibitions and obligations are not to be picked out by the logical feature of being universal in form, but "because the action is a necessary part of a way of life and ideal of conduct. The principal and proximate grounds for claiming that the action must, or must not, be performed are to be found in the characterization of the action offered within the prescription; and if the argument is pressed further, first a virtue or vice and then a whole way of life will have to be described."[47]

Frankena is right to insist that our ability to offer public reasons for our behavior is fundamental to the moral life. But it is not clear that such reasons only work within the context of an abstractly constructed ethics of obligation. Indeed, our obligations make sense only as they are part of ways of life, both communal and individual. In effect this means that we need neither an "ethics of obligation" or an "ethics of virtue" as if those were discrete alternatives. "Obligation" and "virtue" are but reminder terms that help us mark off aspects of our moral existence.

3.4 Obligations and Interests

Even though I cannot hope to do justice to Frankena's meta-ethics, if I am to be fair it is necessary to at least indicate how this aspect of his thought qualifies some of my criticism. Frankena's meta-ethics can be grouped with those that assume that even though the moral point of view may include formal features, it may also involve material considerations.[48] Meta-ethics in certain respects is inherently normative even though this may not imply a morally normative position in the full sense.[49] The very function of morality is to make possible some kind of cooperation or social activity between human beings. Morality rests on the wager that the rational and social aspects of man's existence will coincide.[50] It may well be, moreover, that the current stress on universalizability as the necessary condition of morality is derivative from this fundamental social concern.[51]

In his very important and unfortunately not well-known paper, "Ought and Is Once More," Frankena[52] argues there is not a fundamental rational problem of moving from is to ought in certain contexts once it is realized that "Normative discourse just *is* the appropriate discourse in which to express oneself when one is taking some conative point of view and apprehends facts relevant to it." If one has an interest and believes that certain relevant facts obtain, "then one may rationally and justifiably, at least in principle, proceed to a normative conclusion, even if the inference is not strictly according to *logical* Hoyle."[53] There may be no *logical* way of going from Is to Ought, but it is perfectly reasonable to move from Is to Ought when we have an operative concern or interest.[54]

Frankena[55] argues further that this is not just the characteristic of some uses of ought, but that "all of our Oughts, even those we sometimes use as premises, are generated by or accepted in the presence of some concern or interest in confrontation with some comprehension of fact." Thus, even though it may be that "ought" can be defined, such a definition is really a crystallization of an attitude or interest. Therefore what the definist must keep in mind while rejoicing in this little victory is what really mediates "the inference from Is to Ought or from Fact to Value would not be the definition but the underlying commitment."[56] Frankena is indicating that our moral language is grammatically self-involving, which is essentially my own view.

Frankena helps demonstrate why there can be no easy separation of an ethics of obligation from that of virtue. For what are the virtues but trained interests and commitments for a way of life? The difference between Frankena and myself does not necessarily focus on the interdependence of virtue and obligation, but perhaps in my willingness to entertain a larger range of interests as moral interests.

3.5 Interests, Seeing and "Rationality"

Even though Frankena admits that obligations are correlatives of "interests," not any interests will do; they must be the interests of a "rational" man. Thus the "inference" from Is to Ought is justified only if "any rational being who shares the same concern or point of view will accept them.''[57] Frankena's ''naturalism'' is therefore a rather special kind. ''Right'' is to be understood ''by reference to the concept of 'rationality' which is also involved in the definition of 'true,' not by reference to notions like 'being an object of interest,' 'being demanded by society,' or even 'being in accordance with the will of God.' ''[58]

But the crucial question is how we are to identify this ''rational being'' separated from the interests that make such rationality morally intelligible. Moreover, Frankena must supply us with an epistemology that would make sense of the use of ''true'' when separated from all human interest. I suspect he can meet neither of these demands.

Frankena's position makes sense only if he holds to the Kantian tradition in which a highly specialized sense of ''rationality'' is made the necessary condition of morality. But I think Frankena's analysis of ought language indicates that our ''rationality'' is as dependent on our having the proper virtues as our virtues are dependent on the activity of practical reason. It is no easy task simply to apprehend the ''facts'' truly, for as Frankena rightly observes, our ''facts'' are always determined by our interests. The moral task is to learn to see honestly; such seeing does not come just by looking, but presupposes a steady training in the virtue of humility. To be moral involves being rational, but just as basically it requires us to be humble.[59]

I cannot adequately defend this rather extraordinary claim in this paper. I am not, however, arguing that humility is simply required along with reason for the moral life. Rather, I am suggesting that reason itself requires humility if it is to know at all. The basis for such a claim rests on what I suspect is a fundamental difference between Frankena's and my own view of man. For while I think his analysis of how interests mediate the transition from is to ought is unassailable, he assumes far too readily that men will have the proper interests, that is, that they will want to know the truth or recognize the ''facts.''

Contrary to this, I assume that if we can we will avoid the ''facts.'' Our obligations are correlative to the world we see, but our seeing is inherently perverted by our inveterate tendency to self-deception.[60] To be ''rational'' requires the humility to see the world truthfully, since the world always comes as a challenge to our prideful assumption that we wish to know the ''facts.'' The significance of virtue is clear once we understand that the moral life involves not just what we ought to do, but how we see the world at all.

If I am right that Frankena and I have these quite different assumptions, I am not sure how to go on and I am unclear how such disputes can be resolved. Moreover, even if Frankena and I came to agreement on some of the issues concerning the relation of virtue and obligation, wide areas of disagreement might remain. For our disagreement finally involves basic assumptions about what constitutes the moral life and the corresponding task of ethics.

3.6   *The Institution of Morality and the Relation of Morality to Religion*

Frankena's concern to save "rationality" from dependence on the interests of the self involves his attempt to maintain what he calls the "institution of morality." Moral philosophy is "an attempt to understand what morality is, meaning by 'morality' not the quality of conduct which is opposed to immorality but what Butler so nicely refers to as 'the moral institution of life.' The current endeavor is not to promote certain moral goals or principles, or to clarify only such words as 'right' and 'ought'; but rather to grasp the nature of morality itself, compared with law, religion, or science."[61]

The concern to maintain the "moral institution of life" is exactly what is at stake in elevating the ethics of obligation to "morality" and relegating virtues and ideals to a secondary sense of "moral." For it is assumed that an ethics of obligation could provide the standpoint needed to establish the independence of moral discourse from all the relativities of human interests and commitments save one—the interests of being rational.

The Kantian tradition has rightly felt that obligation language was the most promising way to establish the independence of morality from other human activities. Clearly there are contexts in which we say "I ought to do X," or "you ought to do X" regardless of our or others' interests or desires. Yet this tradition fails to see that such uses of ought presuppose some interests that are not rational in the strict meaning of that term. For to use ought in that manner presupposes the interest of the community to encourage its members to be one way rather than another. Communities can, do and should isolate some actions so important to their own life that they can require their members to conform regardless of their interests or dispositions. These actions may well involve more than just what is necessary for the community to survive, even though current ethical theory tends to associate the language of obligation with defensive ethics. It is, however, unwarranted to declare this aspect of our moral existence to be the whole of morality in distinction to the virtues and ideals we know to be essential to being humane. To do so places ethical reflection too much at the service of the moral judge whose interests are what are minimally required for the functioning of society. Ethics must also be concerned with suggesting those images, virtues and ideals that encourage human flourishing.

The implications of this argument for the relation of religion and morality can only be mentioned. Even though Frankena's analysis of the relation of religion and morality primarily has been concerned with the logical difficulty of moving from descriptive to evaluative propositions, he also has had a moral reason to deny that morality could have a strong relation with religion. His concern to preserve the "institution of morality" serves the moral purpose of holding out the possibility that men can reach consensus on moral grounds, i.e., in terms of what they ought to do. Thus he says, "If morality is dependent on religion, then we cannot hope to solve our problems, or resolve our difficulties of opinion about them, unless and insofar as we can achieve agreement and certainty in religion (not a lively hope); but, if it is not entirely dependent on religion, then we can expect to solve at least some of them by the use of empirical and historical inquiries of a publicly available and testable   kind (inquiries that are improving in quality and scope)."[62]

However, once it is admitted that there can be no easy separation of our duties from our interests (virtues), then the claims of the different religions take on significant moral importance. Not in the sense that the religious beliefs help us to do our duties that we know on independent grounds, but rather that religious beliefs provide a schooling for our dispositions and inter- ests that help us understand what our obligations should be. I am aware that this makes the business of ethics a good deal more messy, but at the same time I think it makes it a good deal more interesting.[63]

3. Natural Law, Tragedy and Theological Ethics

1. Natural Law and Theological Ethics

Recent theological discussions of natural law have concerned two interdependent, but separable, sets of issues. The more prominent issues have been centered around questions of the status of norms and/or absolutes. Associated with, and often confusing, these questions has been the attack on the "past, Roman Catholic, text-book approach to moral theology."[1] The arguments surrounding this set of issues have often been muddled and hopelessly confusing attempts to come up with something called a "dynamic theory of natural law."[2] For example, it is by no means clear how or why questions of the status and types of moral norms and principles are intrinsically tied to natural law.[3] Moreover, what the questions mean or whether the answers to them should be or are central to the business of Christian ethics has not been convincingly demonstrated.

However, natural law, in traditional and recent discussions, has also provided the context for raising the question of the status and truthfulness of the convictions[4] peculiar to Christians, and the relation of those convictions to the form of the moral life of others not sharing those convictions. "Natural law" thus occasions basic methodological issues for theological ethics—namely, what is the form and status of "natural morality" and how does the relation of "natural morality" to Christian convictions help us to know better what it means to claim that such convictions are true.

Many theologians in the name of natural law argue that Christian theology has a stake in the existence of an independent and objective realm of morality. On this presumption the theological task seems to entail trying to locate what all men, Christian and non-Christian, morally share in common.[5] When this search is undertaken under the banner of "natural law," it tends to carry with it the assumption that whatever the content such a shared morality may have, formally it will have a law-like quality. This presumption supplies the con-

necting link between the notion of a common morality and the concern with
the status of moral norms and the proper form of moral theology.

1.1   The Argument in Summary

In this essay I will argue that Christian ethics theologically does not have a
stake in "natural law" understood as an independent and sufficient morality.
In this respect the phrase "natural law" tends to be misleading, as the analogy
with law tends to associate morality with external and minimalistic norms that
Christians can share with all men. Such a view of the moral life makes it extremely difficult to say how grace transforms, reorientates or fulfills natural
law. In contrast to this I will argue that natural morality is best understood not
as a form of law, but rather as the cluster of roles, relations and actions the
agent must order and form to have a character appropriate to the limits
and possibilities of our existence.

Moreover, I will argue that "reason" is not the essence of man, as has been
argued in some natural law theories, but rather that which lays bare and scores
our roles and relationships befitting our nature (agency) as social creatures.
Even though such an ordering is indispensable it will fail, as the basic virtues
of honesty and faithfulness require an ordering beyond what they can supply
in themselves. The necessity to continue to order our lives and actions without
compartmentalizing our behavior and without achieving premature and self-
deceiving synthesis requires a story of forgiveness offered in the cross. Thus,
the "natural moral life" to be lived truly requires the kind of orientation of
character found in the story[6] through which we Christians learn to know and
be like God.

1.2   "Natural Morality" and the Christian

Before developing my positive argument, it will help clarify the problem
central to this essay if I illustrate the kind of difficulties involved in recent
attempts to reinterpret natural law theologically. In contemporary theology we
find statements such as this: "There is no such thing as a natural law existen-
tially separable from the law of Christ, and there never was. There is only
Christian morality, not a natural and a Christian morality."[7] Or: "Natural law
is not really natural; it enters completely into the supernatural economy of
salvation which takes place through the grace of Christ. Joseph Fuchs rightly
says that 'Christ has redeemed the natural law. . . . Natural law does not exist
apart from the grace of Christ.'"[8] McCormick suggests that such claims at
least mean: (1) that natural institutions have a place in Christ's kingdom; (2)

that observance of natural law, since it is a part of the law of Christ, is a means to salvation; and (3) that the good acts of nonbelievers are often or at least potentially performed out of a believing, a Christian love.[9]

Bruno Schüller argues forcefully that "a believer can only hear and understand the message of Christ because he understands and expresses himself as a moral being prior to God's words of revelation. The creator first confronts man with his will in the *lex naturae,* thus making man a possible 'hearer of the word.' Natural moral law is man's *potentia obedientialis* for *lex gratiae.*"[10] Schüller, with rather extraordinary confidence, asserts everyone can see that morality equals love of God, neighbor, and enemy. Therefore the only difference between Christian ethics and non-Christian morality is on the "ontological" level.[11]

All this may seem attractive, but it is extremely unclear what is being said. For natural law is affirmed as being sufficient and yet it can be such only if it is not natural. And we are told that natural law is not separable from Christian morality and yet it can and should be obeyed by those not Christian; or that Christ has "redeemed" the natural law yet the observance of the natural law is in some way tied essentially to the Christian life even when the observance is not qualified in any way by Christian convictions. It is certainly correct to say that the Christian moral life is a natural law ethic inasmuch as Christians claim such a life brings all men to their fullest potential. That is right as a formula, but as an analysis it begs all the issues by redescribing "natural law" as another way to say "Christian."

I fear that Protestant theologians with their much stronger stress on the sinfulness of man have not provided any more clarity. For example, Paul Ramsey defends "natural law," but argues that "Christ must transform the natural law" before it is properly Christian. Thus even though there is some virtue in man's ordinary moral decisions, "no moral judgment is sufficient by nature alone, without in one way or another the saving and transforming power of the *agape* of Christ."[12] Or in the language of justice, the good and evil tendencies in every moral decision suggest ethics cannot be based on reason alone or natural justice. Instead, love must "interpenetrate and invigorate justice at every point."[13] N. H. G. Robinson argues in a similar vein when he says, "For the theological interpretation of morality, the moral continues to stand upon its own feet, to shine by its own light, the mystery of its uniqueness is not denied; but it is seen as a pervasive aspect of an even larger mystery, the mystery of God the creator."[14] Or again, "Christian morality may be a radical reorientation of natural morality, but no less it is of natural morality that it is both the fulfillment and the reorientation."[15]

Though I have sympathy with these positions we have little idea how such words as "transformation," "interpenetrate," "invigorates," "pervasive aspect of larger mystery," "reorientation" and "fulfillment" work. Until

these words and phrases are specified the claims concerning the relation of
Christian morality and natural morality will remain vague and even worse,
uninteresting.

1.3 *"Law," "Virtue" and the Christian Life*

In order to show better how Christian convictions may "transform" natural
morality, I will offer an account of natural morality that borrows more from
the language of virtue than that of law.[16] By doing so I do not mean to deny
the law-like quality of much of our moral existence (especially as this is often
associated with the language of obligation[17]), but rather to remind us that the
moral life also involves the kind of people we should be, the kind of virtues
and character we should have. For when this is forgotten it becomes difficult to make sense out of the kind of claims Christians have wanted to
make about how their convictions form their moral existence.[18]

This is not to deny that much could be made, if a natural law enthusiast so
desired, of how some of the recent "thin" interpretations of morality (Rawls,
Gert, Hare) might be taken as a restatement of what is minimally required of
us as rational creatures. This is especially the case if you think the primary
concern of natural law should be to insure the objectivity of moral rules and
arguments—that is, secure moral judgments from the ambiguities and limitations of history. I will try to show, however, that natural law, when construed
in terms of the virtues necessary to form and secure our social existence,
involves a more complex and richer view of the moral life than these "thin"
theories can provide.[19]

Put briefly, my thesis is that Christian ethics, or better, the language of the
Gospel, suggests the way the moral virtues must be formed if we are to live in
a truthful and nondestructive way. In traditional language the moral virtues
must be formed and given direction in man's character through charity. But
charity does not require the sentimental attempt to go beyond justice as utilitarians would have us believe. Rather, the "old morality" was always right
about this—the new law does not overturn the old law, it can only help you
live with it.

As Peter Geach has argued, knowledge of God is not a prerequisite to our
having *any* moral knowledge. Thus, those that argue that "morality" is not
dependent on religion are at least partly right.[20] But Geach argues further that
the ability to see that we must not do evil that good may come is a correlative
to a certain conception and attitude toward God. Geach does not make clear if
this is a necessary relation or whether one might hold on other grounds than
belief in God that you should not do evil that good may come. I will argue
below that though there is no necessary relation between Christianity and the

"moral" life, the convictions that Christians hold provide them with the skills necessary for the ordering of the moral virtues in a truthful manner, especially as those virtues require us to face moral tragedy.

2. Natural Law: A Constructive Interpretation

For many, Aquinas' "Treatise on Law" (*Summa Theologica,* Qa. 90–108) is the necessary point of origin for thought about natural law. Some are even more restrictive and concentrate only on questions 90–97 of the "Treatise on Law."[21] Questions 98–108, which deal with the old and new laws, are viewed as interesting but dispensable theological ramblings. But this renders Aquinas' reflection on natural law unintelligible, for Aquinas did not discuss natural law in order to supply an "objective" account of natural morality, but rather because he needed a principle of interpretation that would allow him to distinguish the various kinds of precepts found in scripture.[22]

However, one should stress that concentration, even on the full "Treatise on Law" as the statement of Aquinas' analysis of natural law, runs the danger of misinterpretation. For the "Treatise on Law" must be placed within Aquinas' attempt to develop an account of human activity as formed by the virtues. Natural law, like grace, is but the "external principle" of the more fundamental question of man's proper end and activity. It is my contention, therefore, if we are to be faithful to Aquinas, natural law is best discussed in terms of how we are able to find a center for our lives amid the many powers, relations, and roles that lay claim to us.

2.1   The Roles of Men and the Role of Man

Most of our obligations and virtues are role-dependent. In fact, the standards we wish ourselves to be judged by are primarily determined by the roles with which we most intimately identify. Thus, to describe or evaluate our lives always involves judgments about our performance as fathers, lawyers, administrators, mothers, and so on. Bernard Williams has reminded us, however, that while standards may be welded to roles, roles are not logically welded to men. "Through his consciousness of a given title and his relation to it, a man may refuse to make those standards the determinants of his life."[23]

The processes through which we dissociate ourselves from our roles are endless, but it is worth highlighting some of them. Many roles, of course, are simply too limited or not prestigious enough to allow for substantial identification with the self—e.g., a service station attendant or theologian. Or a man may come to dissociate himself from a role, which he had previously completely accepted because he cannot bring himself to do something which he is expected to do in that role.[24] Primary and affective relationships, e.g., friendship, love, husband, son, offer some leverage on our roles, for these commitments, thought quite role-determined themselves, prevent complete identification with the more purposive roles that dominate much of our lives.

Each of these examples suggests that basic to our dissociation from our roles is the inevitable conflict between roles and the expectations they establish in others. Thus, we are forced to set priorities between roles, giving time to one rather than to another, identifying with one in certain contexts and another in other situations, or holding mutually incompatible demands in uneasy harmony. As men we must play many different parts not only successively, but at the same time. This fact makes it difficult to think of ourselves merely as the incumbent of any one role.

Robert Lifton has suggested that the ability of people today to shift roles is a crucial factor in understanding the contemporary context. For men genuinely seem able to live with no primary or fundamental sense of self. Rather, we are ''Protean Men'' who have the ability to move easily from one antithetical role to another without experiencing any fundamental displacement of the self. ''The Protean style of self-process is characterized by an interminable series of experiments and explorations, some shallow, some profound, each of which can readily be abandoned in favor of still new, psychological quests. This pattern resembles, in many ways, what Erik Erikson has called 'identity diffusion' or 'identity confusion' and the impaired psychological functioning which those terms suggest can be very much present. But I want to stress that this Protean style is by no means pathological as such, and in fact may be one of the functional patterns necessary to life in our times.''[25]

I am not concerned to defend or attack Lifton's analysis, but I am sure the condition he describes provides the occasion to ask whether there is a role that helps us set priorities, determine the limits of, and discover the appropriate context of our various roles. For surely, just as traditional natural law arguments have insisted, amidst the welter of our lives there is something that marks man's ability to determine his roles as his own. As Bernard Williams suggests:

> If there were some title or role with which standards were necessarily connected and which, by necessity, a man could not fail to have, nor dissociate himself from, then there would be some standards which a man would have to recognize as determinants of his life, at least on pain of failing to have any consciousness at all of what he was. There is certainly one 'title'—for good reason, we can scarcely speak here of a 'role'—which is necessarily inalienable, and that is the title of 'man' itself. So it is a central question of whether 'man' is a concept which itself provides standards of assessment and excellence as a man; for if it does it seems it must be our standard.[26]

2.2 *Rationality as the "Mark" of Man*

It has been the natural assumption that if such standards are to be derived simply from our being men, they will surely have to do with our most distinguishing mark, our highest capacity. Thus, "rationality" or "intelligence" is taken to be not only a descriptive capability of man, but the standard that provides the basic goals and criteria for a man to allocate and form his other roles. The good man is the man who carries out the function of being human, which is to be "rational."

Even though I have strong sympathies with aspects of the tradition that emphasizes "rationality" as the role of man, I think this emphasis as *the* role of man is misleading.[27] For if one looks at what Aristotle or Aquinas means by "rationality" it becomes apparent that "reason" is not easily abstracted as the "good" of man apart from other characteristics or virtues. Thus, as Aristotle says:

> There exists a capacity called "cleverness," which is the power to perform those steps which are conducive to a goal we have set for ourselves and to attain that goal. If the goal is noble, cleverness deserves praise; if the goal is base, cleverness is knavery. That is why men of practical wisdom are often described as "clever" and "knavish." But in fact this capacity (alone) is not practical wisdom, although practical wisdom does not exist without it. Without virtue or excellence, this eye of the soul (intelligence) does not acquire the characteristics of practical wisdom. Hence, it is clear that a man cannot have practical wisdom unless he is good.[28]

Moreover "rationality" as the "characteristic" or "essence" of man involves an ambiguity not easily resolved. For "rationality" is assumed to be not only a necessary feature of the human condition, but also an ideal that gives direction and scores our varied activities and roles.[29] If the former is emphasized, "morality" tends to be understood as a set of minimal negative prohibitions that are derived from man's "nature";[30] if the latter, "morality" includes matters that seem clearly to go beyond what we think essential to man *qua* man. Yet both these "moralities" are said to be required by natural law so far as man is "rational." There seems to be no satisfactory way of harmonizing these claims as long as "reason" is taken as the role of man that gives normative direction to his being.

My basic difficulty with "rationality" as the "mark" of man, however, is that when reason is abstracted from the other goods that enhance our lives it becomes a technical instrument for man's attempt to secure survival. Reason thus often becomes wedded to self-interest as the tool to secure my existence against others. At best practical reason takes the form of instrumental calculation to secure the least harm for the greatest number. Morality is modified self-interest as we care for the other only so far as it rationally is in our self-interest to try to secure the survival of as many of our fellows as possible.[31]

Such a view of "reason" always is in danger of ideological perversion, especially as it takes the form of a criterion of the "justice" of a social system.[32] For in fact the way we "reason" to score the diverse roles of our lives has little to do with "calculation" of results. None live for survival as an end in itself, but rather we live for goods that make survival worthwhile. Reason is not separable from the ways of life that form our behavior to be one way rather than another. "What we survive *as* is more important than whether we survive in the simple sense of physical persistence; and thus too, since we must all die, it has always seemed important to those that have lived to the fullest extent of their capacities that somehow this feature of their life be significantly incorporated into a rationally principled action or series of action."[33] Reason is not a passive faculty for the apprehension of "reality," "for practical truth does not consist in the mind's conformity to what is but in its conformity with the rectified appetite," i.e., an appetite formed by virtues worthy of man.[34]

2.3 *Action, Reason and Sociality*

Therefore, appeals to natural law, "human nature" or "reason" are best understood not as metaphysical descriptions necessary to ground ethical judgments, but rather value-laden notions that remind us of how we should best score and order our roles in the world.[35] To claim humanity is not just to assume a membership in the biological class *homo sapiens,* but rather it is an attempt to see ourselves as having a social role in the universe as a member of a species. As Herbert McCabe has pointed out, to be told:

> "This belongs to the species of panther" is a remark different from, and more informative than "this is a panther." To be told that it belongs to a species is to be told not that there are others like it but that part of what this panther is is to be a fragment of a larger whole. It is to be told that part of its behaviour is to be explained by the requirements of this larger whole. Not to know that the panther belongs to a species would be not to know something about this individual panther; membership in the species is part of what it means for the panther to be itself. It is a consequence of this that when its behaviour is influenced by its membership of the species, it is not suffering violence from the outside. In a parallel way, when a man obeys the law of his "species," the natural law, he is being true to a depth within himself, and that to act contrary to this law is to violate himself at his center.[36]

The question of the role of man *qua* man is, therefore, a question primarily designed to remind us that not all the ways that humans can live are equally humane. Appeals to natural law suggest "that morality need not only be a matter either of following the *mores* or of freely choosing how to live and seeing social morality as *mauvaise foi*. It can also be a matter of *discovering* how it is possible for people to live together in ways which lead to an increasing capacity for mutual trust and moral growth."[37] Once this is presupposed it makes sense to emphasize our rational ability as skills crucial to our attempt to build humane communities.

Reason, so understood, is but an aspect of our fundamental ability to act. As Charles Fried reminds us, "natural law is a theory of action,"[38] for to be a man is to act rather than be acted upon.[39] To say that we are rational is to claim that as agents we can deliberate and plan our behavior; but moreover, we *ought* so to act, in the sense that as social creatures not to do so is to be less than what we could be, for only by doing what we ought can we be what we are.[40] In contrast to the sense of rationality criticized above, this understanding of "reason" is not committed to the idea that there is only one way to be rational—the variety of our rational activities is only limited by the language of our communities.[41]

This sense of "rationality" does not commit us to specifying any one end or project for man. For there to be a "role" that organizes our various "roles" does not mean that we must have one purpose or end that dominates all others, but only that we must have a story that gives direction to our character. Aristotle's emphasis on happiness as the last end of man is misleading in this respect. For happiness is not an end that can be striven for, but rather is a characteristic that is simply commensurate with a life well lived.[42] *Eudaimonia* is but a name for a set of virtuous activities,[43] and thus the crucial question is what gives order to this set.[44]

2.4 Natural Law, Sociality and Promise Keeping

"Rationality," therefore, names our ability to act and to give reasons for our actions. Thus, to speak of reason but reminds us of our more fundamental commitment to living in concert with the powers within us and the persons around us. The necessity of offering reasons for our actions is not to meet some formal demand of "morality" or "rationality," but rather it is an attempt to gesture our basic indebtedness to the institutions that have formed us and the persons with whom we travel and work. "If we were formed to select the principle that supports and infuses all human aspirations we would find it in the objective of maintaining communication with our fellows. Communication is something more than staying alive. It is a way of being alive."[45] Natural law is therefore not based on a view of the "nature" of man abstracted from his social context, but rather, as Calvin emphasized, the natural law is but a reminder that "to be human is to order life cooperatively."[46]

When natural law is understood in this manner, promise keeping becomes the central paradigm for the moral life. The necessity to give reasons for what we do is our attempt to fulfill the promissory relation that pertains between us. To be sure, no explicit "promise" has been made, but our explicit "promises" remind us how much of our life is dependent on implicit expectations of trust and faithfulness.[47] As Knud Lögstrup suggests:

> It is a characteristic of human life that we naturally trust one another. This is true not only in the case of persons who are well acquainted with one another but also in the case of utter strangers. Only because of some special circumstance do we ever distrust a stranger in advance. Perhaps some informer has destroyed the natural trust which people spontaneously have toward one another, so that their relationship becomes oppressive and strained. Under normal circumstances, however, we accept the stranger's word and do not mistrust him until we have some particular reason to do so. We never suspect a person of falsehood until after we have caught him in a lie. If we enter into a conversation on the train with a person whom we have never met before and about whom we know absolutely nothing, we assume that what he says is true and do not become suspicious of him unless he begins to indulge in wild exaggerations. Nor do we normally assume a person to be a thief; not until he conducts himself in a suspicious manner do we begin to suspect him. Initially we believe one another's word; initially we trust one another. This may indeed seem strange, but it is part of what it means to be human. Human life could hardly exist if it were otherwise. We would simply not be able to live; our life would be impaired and wither away if we were in advance to distrust one another, if we were to suspect the other of thievery and falsehood from the very outset.[48]

Promising as a characteristic of our lives rather than simply a discrete institution places heavy demands on our ability to use language.[49] Our commitment to truth, to saying what is, is a form of our commitment to maintain the trust between ourselves. "The use of language implies a commitment as much as life in society does—a commitment to communicate, i.e., to use that language in a way that others may understand if they too are users of that language; i.e., to use that language properly. Thus, Jones has an obligation to follow through on that promise he made to Smith, and so does an anarchist who opposes the whole institution of promising—the obligation is built into the language, which is built into the institution, and the institution is built into nature by the fact that man is a potential, i.e., an institutional, animal."[50]

Moreover, promising reveals the basis for our recognition and necessary respect for the other. "Here we see the special place of the capacity for sociability in human nature, sociability being the capacity of human persons to use their own powers of freedom and rationality to recognize the same powers in others and to make the full use in their own acts of those powers as exemplified in the acts of others."[51] It is on this basis that natural law has rightly been thought to provide grounds for claims of moral equality.[52] Such claims I am sure can be further specified by rules of fair play that are essential for the moral life of a society. These rules, however, will appear quite different within different cultural contexts.[53] Thus, how the Christian moral life is understood and related materially to non-Christian morality will necessarily differ from one society to another.

However, it would be a mistake to take the derivation of such rules to be the primary function of natural law. For natural law as the search for a center that provides men a way to order their various roles is more a matter of the virtues than the rules. As Albert Jonsen suggests:

the natural law is not a set of rules, ordering in detail the life of man. It is first a consideration of the radical exigencies of the human person in the human community, then a consequent consideration about the form of human behavior which will promote these potentialities. Even these consequent considerations are not exactly rules. They are rather what we used to call by that now discredited Victorian word, virtues. Thus, natural law prescribes the virtue of "honesty" as the form of life preservative of self-reflective consciousness. It is another step, a rather more complicated one, to proceed from this to a rule about "truth-telling." Likewise, natural law prescribes the virtue of fidelity as the form of life preservative of self-engaging commitment. One must go into many details to work out rules of promise-keeping, contract, etc.[54]

There can be no shortcut for how such "details" are worked out, as they must be hewn from the common life of a people. Without a tradition there is no articulation of the natural law,[55] but equally the tradition may prescribe matters that are incumbent on the agent which go beyond what is required for survival.

3. Natural Law and the Christian Life

It still remains for me to show how this understanding of natural morality displays *how* Christian convictions shape and give form to the moral life. I have construed natural morality primarily in terms of the necessity of people to find the limits and order among the various rules we embody. I have suggested that the virtues of honesty and faithfulness provide the form and direction for our orientation as people who are social beings. In other words, the boundaries of our roles, professional, familial, or interpersonal, are set by how well they serve the moral prerequisites incumbent on us as social beings.

But the virtues of honesty and faithfulness are not always compatible. We sometimes find that if we are to be honest to one we must be unfaithful to another. For honesty is a hard virtue, as it must destroy our own and others' deceptions. Thus, even though honesty and faithfulness are basic to our lives, they are not sufficient to provide the kind of order to our lives necessary to sustain their own enterprise over our lives. Honesty and faithfulness require more than themselves if they are to be the guiding stars of our lives.

This "something more" is not necessarily Christian convictions, for other convictions also lay claim to how honesty and virtue can be sustained. Yet Christians can rightly claim that they have found the Christian story of forgiveness releases them to develop the skills needed to take up honesty and faithfulness as lifetime projects. For forgiveness provides the assurance that the truth is bounded by God's grace. We can thus have the confidence to let truth empower our lives as a way of life that directs all our endeavors. Put this way it is clear that the natural morality is indeed natural; that is, Christian convictions may add nothing to honesty or faithfulness. Yet each requires formation by convictions beyond their own range if we are to know how to embody them in our lives. What grace "transforms," "interpenetrates," "reorientates," is not the virtues themselves, but rather the self—our character—that must be formed to bear the heavy demands of a life truthfully and faithfully lived.

I suspect that this is what Augustine was trying to suggest when he argued that even the virtues which the soul "seems to itself to possess, and by which it restrains the body and the vices that it may obtain and keep what it desires, are rather vices than virtues so long as there is no reference to God in the matter."[56] The "reference to God" does not change the form of the individual virtues, but rather orders them into an orientation to man's primary role. Thus:

> temperance is love giving itself entirely to that which is loved; fortitude is readily bearing all things for the sake of the loved object; justice is love serving only the loved object, and therefore ruling rightly; prudence is love distinguishing with sagacity between what hinders it and what helps it. The object of this love is not anything, but only God, the chief good, the highest wisdom, the perfect harmony. So we may express the definition thus: that temperance is love keeping itself entire and incorrupt for God; fortitude is love bearing everything readily for the sake of God; justice is love serving God only, and therefore ruling well all else, as subjects to man; prudence is love making a right distinction between what helps it towards God and what might hinder it.[57]

It is probably the better part of wisdom to end on this homiletical note, but I wish to make a few final remarks in hopes of clarifying my position. I argued above that survival is not and cannot be a proper end for the moral life. This rather obvious and perhaps platitudinous assertion has ramifications which are seldom appreciated. For if the end of life is not survival, then the moral problem is how and under what condition would we be willing to die and let others die. For if we have rightly scored our life according to the virtues demanded by our sociality, then we must be willing to die or have others die rather than act contrary to those virtues.

Fried's discussion of *Regina v. Dudley and Stevens* is extremely illustrative in this respect. For contrary to the utilitarian assumption that all that matters is to save as many lives as possible, Fried correctly maintains that more important is "how the act was done, how the lives were saved" or lost. Thus, in *Dudley and Stevens* the question is "not simply the one of numerical survival but the quality of the act by which survival is purchased."[58] What was done on the lifeboat was wrong, not simply because procedures were not used that insured the fairness of the choice of survivors, but because survival itself was taken as overriding the value of trust that makes life morally a worthy goal.

It is not my purpose here to argue whether lots should have been drawn, or, failing to get volunteers, whether all should have been willing to die,[59] but rather to point out that this is a paradigm example of the nature of our existence. For as Fried argues, "Every act of an entity changes the total circumstances in which other entities must act and thus every act of a human agent impinges on other human agents."[60] To live morally thus means that we must necessarily be willing to risk our own and others' lives for those values we find necessary to maintain our life together. In certain crucial cases, such as the lifeboat case, we must be willing to let ourselves and others die rather than to act against these goods.[61] As stated in the *Mishnah Sanhedrin* (4:15), "For this reason was one single man created: to teach you that anyone who destroys a single life is as though he destroyed the whole of mankind; and anyone who preserves a single life is as though he preserved the whole of mankind."

Some think that cases where life itself must be chosen raise no problems, since the distinction between direct and indirect may be invoked. This distinction is an attempt to let us have our moral commitments without willing the tragedies that they necessarily involve. For the theist to admit moral tragedy[62] seems to impugn the goodness of God's intentions, as we assume that a good God could create a world where positive moral goods would not conflict. For the rationalist moral tragedy makes moral argument too tentative and dependent on *a priori* commitments. Yet if I am right, there is no way to avoid admitting that to be moral necessarily requires us to be faithful to our commitments even though those same commitments require our own and others' lives.[63] The problem with the distinction between direct-indirect is not that it fails to make logical sense,[64] but that it gives us the illusion that we can be honest and faithful without sacrifice.

Once this kind of issue is faced, I think we have at least located the kind of problem that has led Christians to argue that "natural law" was incomplete. The demands of living morally are hard, for the wish to be and do good invites self-deceiving explanations for those tragedies we cannot morally prevent. We do not wish to face the truth that we live in a world where honesty and faithfulness do not always lead to good results and consequences, but sometimes to tragic choices.[65] It is only when we admit this and learn to embody it in our lives that we can begin to understand why Christian ethics is not basically an ethics of principle, but rather a story of a God who is found most vividly in the past and continuing history of Israel and in the form of the Cross. Adherence to such a God does not change what it means ideally to act in this life, but it may help us know how to live such a life without deception.[66]

4. Story and Theology

1. The Theological Use of Story

We all love a good story. For example, if I had begun this essay with the phrase, "I would like to begin by telling you a story," I would have your attention much more than I do now. A story commands our attention much more than a lecture about stories. We often remember the stories we heard in a lecture or a sermon even though we cannot remember why they were told in the first place.

The power of stories to command our attention has opened up a fruitful line of investigation for theological reflection. For it is obvious that whatever else it is the message that appears central to the Christian faith is in the form of a story. Perhaps it is possible, therefore, for the Christian story to cash in on the general interest we all seem to have in stories.

Yet this is to put the issue too simply, as some are suggesting that Christian convictions[1] are not accidentally formed in a story but that this is necessarily the case. In other words the fact that we learn about God or Jesus in the form of a story is not sufficient to establish the importance of "story" as essential for the theological task. The argument is not that some theology may be expressed via narrative, but the "stronger suggestion that narrative or story is a means of expression uniquely suited to theology or at least to Christian theology."[2] This does not mean that all theology must itself assume the form of narrative, but rather whatever form theological reflection may take, one of its primary tasks is reminding us of a story. And of course one of the best ways to remind anyone of a story is by telling another story.

Sallie TeSelle puts it well as she asks,

> Why does everyone love a good story and how is story related to theological reflection? The answers to these two questions are, I believe, related. We all love a good story because of the basic narrative quality of human experience; in a sense, any story is about ourselves, and a *good* story is good precisely because somehow it rings true to human life. Human life is not marked by instantaneous rapture and easy solutions. Life is tough. That

71

is hardly a novel thought, but it is nonetheless the backbone in a literal sense—the 'structure'—of a good story. We recognize our own pilgrimages from here to there in a good story; we feel its movement in our bones and know it is 'right.' We love stories, then, because our lives are stories and in the attempts of others to move, temporally and painfully, we recognize our own story. For the Christian, the story of Jesus is *the* story par excellence. That God should be with us in the story of a human life could be seen as a happy accident, but it makes more sense to see it as God's way of always being with human beings *as they are*, as the concrete, temporal beings who have a beginning and an end—who are, in other words, stories themselves.[3]

1.1   Possible Misuses of "Story" in Theology

Now I think that this emphasis on the importance of story as the grammar of theology is very suggestive, but it is important that we get it right. For example, I think that TeSelle rightly suggests that there are or may be important links between biography and autobiography, the narrative element in Scripture, and the narrative quality of "experience." But because we suspect that such links exist does not mean that we understand what kind of connections they are. Moreover, it would be disastrous if this emphasis on the significance of story for theological reflection became a way to avoid the question of how religious convictions or stories may be true or false, i.e., you have your story and we have ours and there is no way to judge the truth of either.

For example, Hans Frei makes the useful suggestion that the gospels are best thought of not as history, but rather realistic narratives, which while "history like," are not history.[4] But this suggestion would be disastrous if it is an attempt to make irrelevant whether Jesus in fact did not exist and act in a way very much like the way he is portrayed in the gospel accounts. For the demand that what Jesus was not be different than how we have come to know him in the gospels is not based on some external demand of historical truth, but rather because the very nature of the story of Jesus itself demands that Jesus be the one who in fact the church said and continues to say he is.

The emphasis on story can also be misleading for the theological task if we take comfort in the argument that a story does not need a "factual" basis in order to be truthful. We know that often fiction is "truer" than history—that Doctorow's *Ragtime* may tell us more about America than many histories of the same period.[5] Or even more radically we are learning that the line between history and fiction may not be as exact as the causal model of historical explanation has led us to believe, for insofar as historical explanation must take the form of narrative it is much more like "fiction" than "science."[6] But even granting that there is a truth to fiction and a fictitious quality to "historical'' truth, it remains to be spelled out how the truth of the story of Jesus on which we stake our lives may or may not be like the truth found in fiction and/or history.

1.2 Story and the Truthfulness of Religious Convictions

To point to the story character of religious convictions may however help us to avoid some of the misleading ways that the religious convictions are often thought to be true or false. For example, questions like does God really exist or did Jesus rise from the grave are sometimes taken as the central questions that determine the truth or falsity of religious convictions. God's existence and Jesus' resurrection are not unimportant convictions for Christians, but it is inappropriate to single them out as *the* issues of religious truth. For the prior question is how the affirmations of God's existence and Jesus' resurrection fit into the story of the kind of God we have come to know in the story of Israel and Jesus. The emphasis on story as the grammatical setting for religious convictions is the attempt to remind us that Christian convictions are not isolatable ''facts,'' but those ''facts'' are part of a story that helps locate what kind of ''fact'' you have at all.[7]

In other words, I am interested in ''story'' and theology not because the narrative form may be a way of avoiding how religious convictions may or may not be true. Instead I hold the more positive view that the story quality of the gospels provides the appropriate context to raise the issue of truth at all. The question of truth must be commensurate with the form and kind of claims that are being made. To emphasize the story character of the gospel is an attempt to suggest that examining the truth of Christian convictions is closely akin to seeing how other kinds of stories form our lives truly or falsely.

Thus story is a way to remind us of the inherently practical character of theological convictions. For Christian convictions are not meant to picture the world. They do not give a primitive metaphysics about how the world is constituted. Rather the gospel is a story that gives you a way of being in the world. Stories, at least the kind of stories I am interested in, are not told to explain as a theory explains, but to involve the agent in a way of life. A theory is meant to help you know the world without changing the world yourself; a story is to help you deal with the world by changing it through changing yourself.

This is the reason, as I have argued elsewhere, that ethics cannot be separated from theology.[8] As Bernard Williams has argued, ''the point of morality is not to mirror the world, but to change it; it is concerned with such things as principles of action, choice, responsibility. The fact that men of equal intelligence, factual knowledge, and so forth, confronted with the same situation, may morally disagree shows something about morality—that (roughly) you cannot pass the moral buck on to how the world is. But that does not show that there is something *wrong* with it.''[9] Neither is it the point of stories to mirror the world of empirical facts, but that does not mean stories do not help us know about the world. It is rather to remind us that the world that we can know about is also the world that includes human activity as part of its facticity. As such, part of the "facts" that are to be known can be known only by having stories that form and thus provide appropriate knowledge of the world. Thus the truth of religious convictions at least involves how the self is formed to rightly know the world as it should be but is not, except as it is subject to divine and human agency.

Thus the emphasis on "story" is not an attempt to rob religious conviction of cognitive significance, but rather to get right the kind of cognitive claims religious convictions involve. To be sure, stories tell you about the world, but how they tell you about the world involves how the self is situated in the world. As Wittgenstein suggested in the *Tractatus:*

> If the good or bad exercise of the will does alter the world, it can alter only the limits of the world, not the facts—not what can be expressed by means of language.
> In short the effect must be that it becomes an altogether different world. It must, so to speak, wax and wane as a whole.
> The world of the happy man is a different one from that of the unhappy man. (6.43)

As yet, these comments, however, remain far too general to be of much help, as I have not yet defined or clarified the meaning of "story." Like the role that "grace" plays in some theologies, "story" is sometimes used as such an inclusive category it tends to be vacuous. As George Stroup has suggested, much of the theology emphasizing the category of story tends to offer a vague description of "story," and then use "it as an excuse, rather than a systematic principle, for the discussion of other themes.''[10] I have no desire to make story a "systematic principle," but Stroup's call for analytical clarity is well-founded. We must turn to the question, "What is a story?"

2.   What Is a Story

Like Augustine trying to understand time, the category of story becomes remarkably elusive as soon as we ask what it is. We all know it when we hear a story, we even know what counts for a good story, but when we go to say what a story is it proves to be hard to get hold of. Perhaps part of our difficulty is that stories have many different forms and functions. Some we listen to because we know the ending, others because we do not know they will end. Sometimes we say, "That is just a story," thereby marking one account off from "what really happened"; but other times we assume that the only way to say "what really happened" is by telling a story, i.e., "Now tell me the real story."

Some stories are short-lived jokes while others come in the form of extended and grand tales. Stories seem to be the glue that binds together such diverse literary enterprises as history, autobiography, biography, novels, folktales and myths. It is not my intention to try to delineate the differences and similarities between these genres of story-telling or to account for the various points of view within a story or from which stories can be told.[11] Nor will I try, as Hans Frei does, to claim that the gospel is closer to realistic narrative and thus non-mythic.[12] Stories can be realistic or mythical and perhaps both at the same time. Rather, I want to try the more modest task of eliciting the characteristics of the concept of story that allows us to say, "That is one," and why we think they are important.

We can begin with the thought that a story at least seems to involve "an imputed pattern of human relationships richer, more throbbing and intense than appearances may actually justify."[13] But it is not just any imputed pattern, but a pattern that takes the form of narrative.[14] For it seems, just as it is necessary in order to distinguish an action from an event that we must be able to ask the question "Why,"[15] so a story must at least elicit the question, "What happens next?"[16]

But exactly the reason we are invited to ask "What happened next?" also reveals an essential aspect of narrative, because narrative is a connection between non-necessary, contingent events. As Lou Mink suggests,

> Surprises and contingencies are the stuff of stories, as of games, yet by virtue of the promised yet open outcomes we are enabled to follow a series of events across their contingent relations and to understand them as leading to an as yet unrevealed conclusion without however necessitating that conclusion. We may follow understandingly what we could not predict or infer. Stories may be followed more or less completely, as a wise old hand at cricket may notice nice details which escape the spectator of average keenness, and there can be no criteria for following completely. But the minimal conditions are the same for all. The features which enable a story to flow and us to follow, then, are the clues to the nature of historical understanding. An historical narrative does not demonstrate the necessity of events but makes them intelligible by unfolding the story which connects their significance.[17]

Stories are thus a necessary form of our knowledge inasmuch as it is only through narrative that we can catch the connections between actions and responses of men that are inherently particular and contingent.[18] The intentional nature of human action is exactly that which creates the space demanding narrative as the necessary form to account for the connection and intelligiblity of our activity. The structure of a particular narrative is not in any exact way the structure of reality, but narrative form is a necessary way of seeing, transforming, and to some extent re-expressing reality true to the form of human action. As the narrator of Doctorow's *Welcome to Hard Times* says, "Really how life gets on is a secret, you only know your memory, and it makes its own time. The real time leads you along and you never know when it happens, the best that can be is come and gone." Thus to describe an action rightly is not to give its causal antecedents, but rather "describing it as a response and therefore as an element in a story. Otherwise it would not even be represented as an action (that is, as intentional and having a meaning for the agent), but as an opaque bit of behavior waiting for its story to be told."[19]

The characteristics that Frei attributes to realistic narrative apply to all stories in this respect. For stories require a narrative depiction in which "characters or individual persons, in their internal depth or subjectivity as well as in their capacity as doers and sufferers of actions or events, are firmly and significantly set in the context of the external environment, natural but more particularly social. Realistic narrative is that kind in which subject and social setting belong together, and characters and external circumstances fitly render each other. Neither character nor circumstances separately, nor yet their interaction, is a shadow of something else more real or more significant. Nor is the one more important than the other in the story. 'What is character but the determination of incident? What is incident but the illustration of character?' asked Henry James."[20] Thus what draws us to stories is not the story, seen as the enumeration of events, but rather the interaction of events and the people that make them. As Scholes and Kellogg suggest, "Quality of mind (as expressed in the language of characterization, motivation, description, and commentary) not plot, is the soul of narrative. Plot is only the indispensable skeleton which, fleshed out with character and incident, provides the necessary clay into which life may be breathed."[21]

A story, thus, is a narrative account that binds events and agents together in an intelligible pattern. We do not tell stories simply because they provide us a more colorful way to say what can be said in a different way, but because there is no other way we can articulate the richness of intentional activity— that is, behavior that is purposeful but not necessary. For as any good novelist knows there is always more involved in any human action than can be said. To tell a story often involves our attempt to make intelligible the muddle of things we have done in order to have a self.

3.   The Indispensability of Stories

Stories are not just a literary genre, therefore, but a form of understanding that is indispensable. As Frei argues about realistic narrative, there is "the indispensability of the narrative shape, including chronological sequence, to the meaning, theme, or subject matter of the story.''[22] In other words stories do not illustrate a meaning, they do not symbolize a meaning, but rather the meaning is embodied in the form of the story itself. Put differently, stories are indispensable if we are to know ourselves; they are not replaceable by some other kind of account.

Let me try to illustrate this point by calling our attention to two different uses of stories that are often confused. The first kind of story is that which is told us to make a point or produce a certain effect (laughter) in such a way that the point or the effect is separable from the story itself. For example, we tell a story about Richard Nixon in order to make the point that politics is a messy business, or the nature of the American society, or to illustrate the moral principle you ought never to lie. Now what is interesting about this is that another story would do just as well to make the point, i.e., here, stories are interchangeable.

Now I suspect that this form of story is paradigmatic for us, namely, we have the idea that all stories are somehow used to make a point that is separable from the story itself. In our everyday life we are often impatient with the story-teller—we want him to get on to the point, not to waste our time with all the embellishments of the story. Stories were for slower times when we did not need to get things done. Or we are taught that stories cannot have to do with truth as truth is truth exactly to the extent that it can be separated from its story or history, that is, we must be able to get the same results even though we are not in the same time or geographical location. The experiment must be separable from the experimenter.

This paradigm of stories is so strong we have tended to forget that our lives are formed by another kind of story, namely, the stories that have no point beyond the story itself. We have instances of this but we often fail to notice them. For example, think about the experience of finishing a novel in which you have been deeply engrossed. Moreover, let's suppose that through reading the novel you gained the skill to articulate a haunting insight that you had intuitively known but had not been able to state with clarity, e.g., no one can love without causing pain. Now as so often happens when we finish a good novel, we want to share the novel and the insight with someone else, but somehow the insight sounds platitudinous separated from the novel itself. (Or in a philosophical context, what is important is not the conclusion but the argument itself.) So in order to rescue the insight you try to tell the novel to your companion, but that does not work either because there is no way in the telling you can capture the subtlety of description. (This I suspect is why the question of the relation of art and morality is so tricky, namely, that the moral insight cannot be separated from the intricacies of the story.) So in desperation we give up trying to tell what we have "learned" from the novel and simply assert that our companion must read the novel to "understand" what we mean.

There is another instance of this kind of experience where we have difficulty separating the point from the story itself. Think for example of what happens when we introduce ourselves to someone. We give our name, birthplace, vocation or profession, some major event of our past—the elements that make up the story of our life. Now I suspect that we would be a little chagrined if after such a telling of our story we were asked, "But what is the point?" The story is the point, for our life cannot be separated from the story. As Steven Crites has suggested, "A man's sense of his own identity seems largely determined by the kind of story which he understands himself to have been enacting through the events of his career, the story of his life."[23] Of course, we could be asked to give the "real" story, namely, our questioner suspects we have been hiding something about who we are and thus asks for a fuller or more accurate story. Notice what you must ask for is not a neutral account of the same story, but rather you must ask for another story.

Now this seems to me to be very significant, for it suggests that there are aspects of our experience that make story unavoidable. I am not suggesting just that we require stories to understand who we are, though we certainly do. As Sallie TeSelle says, "We learn who we are through the stories we embrace as our own—the story of my life is structured by the larger stories (social, political, mythic) in which I understand my personal story to take place."[24] But rather I am suggesting that the mysterious thing we call a self is best understood exactly as a story—a story that has no point but the display of itself for others, but especially for ourselves.

4. Story and the Stories of Self and God

I would not want to claim that stories are necessary for articulating everything about our existence. Some things can be accounted for without appeal to stories, and other kinds of explanations can be substituted for stories in some contexts. But stories are indispensable for those matters that deal with the irreducible particular, that is, that which cannot be other than it is and thus cannot be accounted for by any other. In other words, stories are required by those matters that we can only describe analogically.[25] Our mistakes occur intellectually when we assume that we can give a better account of these particulars than stories can provide, namely, when we try to state the point without the story.[26]

What may be called for is a better story, but what cannot be called for is a literal or perhaps "metaphysical" account that makes the "story" irrelevant. There is no story of stories, i.e., an account that is literal and that thus provides a criterion to say which stories are true or false. All we can do is compare stories to see what they ask of us and the world which we inhabit.

Of particular interest for theological reflection is that story seems to be indispensable in order to express the nature of two such particulars—the self and God. For example, Hannah Arendt has pointed out that to say who someone is, whether that someone be ourselves or another, eludes precise speech. Thus "the moment we want to say *who* somebody is, our very vocabulary leads us astray into saying *what* he is; we get entangled in a description of qualities he necessarily shares with others like him; we begin to describe a type or a 'character' in the old meaning of the word, with the result that his uniqueness escapes us."[27] But she suggests that we can surmount this difficulty through story. "*Who* somebody is or was we can know only by knowing the story of which he is himself the hero—his biography, in other words; everything else we know of him, including the work he may have left behind, tells us only *what* he is or was."[28] What we must know how to do is to spell out in story form that a person is not like a type, but is a proper name. Indeed, a story can and does function like a proper name and vice versa.

Now if this account of the significance of story for the self is correct, it helps us have a sense why it is that story is an essential characteristic of Christian discourse. For like the self, God is a particular agent that can be known only as we know his story. Too often it has been assumed that we can talk of God as if he is a universal, namely, that the grammar of God is like the grammar of trees, towns or persons. But the grammar of God is not that of an indefinite noun, but rather of a proper name. This means God is not a necessary being. Put starkly, God is not a concept, but a name like Stanley Hauerwas.[29]

Thus if we are to learn to speak of God we must learn to speak of him in stories.[30] The crucial question is not whether there is a way of avoiding stories when we speak of God, but which stories best enable us to speak of him and of our relation to him truthfully. It is not sufficient simply to appeal to the stories that we find in the scripture, for they are many and various. But if we cannot appeal to authority, then we seem at a loss, as it is not even clear what kind of question this is, much less how we might proceed to answer it.

5. The Truthfulness of the Stories of God and the Self

A fruitful way to at least begin thinking about this question, or perhaps better to identify what kind of question it is, is to ask what kind of story must I have to speak of myself truthfully. For even if it is correct to say that the self cannot avoid being a story—we are irreducibly story—then the question is how can we know that the story that we are can also be known to be true, true not for anyone else at this point but myself. For we know that too often the story that we identify with—I am an old Texas boy trying to make good—does little to capture the actuality of the story that we are living out.

Put more directly, we often think that a true story is one that provides an accurate statement, a correct description. However, I am suggesting that a true story must be one that helps me to go on, for, as Wittgenstein suggested, to understand is exactly to know how to go on.[31] For when we do not understand, we are afraid, and we tell ourselves stories that protect ourselves from the unknown and foreign—indeed, stories that even deny that there is an unknown or foreign. Thus a true story is one that helps me to uncover the true path that is also the path for me through the unknown and foreign. It is important to note in this sense I cannot make the story true by how I use it, but the story must make me true to its own demands of how the world should be.

For we must remember that the world is not simply waiting to be seen, but we must learn to see by how we insist on seeing it. But our seeing too often is a seeing that is bounded by trying to secure our past achievements. We thus fall inextricably into self-deception.[32] A story that is true must therefore demand that we be true and provide us with the skills to yank us out of our self-deceptions, the main one of which is that we wish to know the truth. It is only on the basis of such a story that we can know how to go on with the courage appropriate to human existence. Put more simply, I am suggesting that "truth is not separable from other measures of value—from consistency, righteousness, justice, happiness, satisfaction."[33]

A true story thus must enable us to know what our engagements have committed us to. For even though our lives must be displayed by stories, our life is not any one story. "Life has no beginnings, middles, or ends; there are meetings, but the start of an affair belongs to the story we tell ourselves later, and there are partings, but final partings only in the story. We could learn to tell stories of our lives from nursery rhymes, or from culture-myths if we had any, but it is from history and fiction that we learn how to tell and to understand complex stories, and how it is that stories answer questions."[34]

But we know how hard it is to find a story that allows us to be truthful with ourselves. For the bulk of us have no central story, we are just bits of many stories. Thus the very story that was truthful yesterday I have learned to use to support a false account today. If this is the case with ourselves, then how are we to know which stories of God are true, misleading, or false?

We are, of course, not without resources, as we have the work of a tradition that has witnessed to the stories that are central to being a people called by God. Moreover, we can look to how the saints have been formed by the stories of God that have made them truthful beings. For at least part of what it means to claim that convictions of Christians are true is that they must produce truthful lives. For if as James McClendon has argued, "Christian beliefs are not so many 'propositions' to be catalogued or juggled like truth-functions in a computer, but are living convictions which give shape to actual lives and actual communities, we open ourselves to the possibility that the only relevant critical examination of Christian beliefs may be one which begins by attending to lived lives. Theology must be at least biography. If by attending to those lives, we find ways of reforming our own theologies, making them more true, more faithful to our ancient vision, more adequate to the age now being born, then we will be justified in that arduous inquiry.''[35]

But then perhaps it is the case that the true stories that we learn of God are those that help us best to know what story we are and should be, that is, that which gives us the courage to go on. Namely, the story that is necessary to know God is the story that is also necessary to know the self, but such knowing is not the passive accomodation to an external object. Rather such a knowing is more like a skill that gives us the ability to know the world as it is and should be—it is a knowing that changes the self. Thus to ask how I am to know which story best helps me know myself or God is in fact two interdependent questions, not in the sense that one is logically necessary for the answer to the other, but rather each is morally necessary to the other if we are to have a story that provides us with the skills to form our lives truthfully.[36]

5. Self-Deception and Autobiography: Reflections on Speer's *Inside the Third Reich*

with David B. Burrell

1. Introduction

This essay brings together two interests: the relationship of philosophy of mind to ethics and the challenge of Auschwitz for persons who intend to be Christian. Any analysis of Speer's autobiography necessarily joins these interests, for *Inside the Third Reich* offers a paradigm illustration of the connection between self-deception and cooperation with murder. The argument structuring this essay shows how our ability to know what we are up to and live authentically depends on our capacity to avoid self-deception. We cannot hope to avoid an inveterate tendency to self-deception, however, unless we work at developing the skills required to articulate the shape of our individual and social engagements, or forms of life. At the heart of such skills lies a practiced eye and ear for the basic images and stories that provide our actions with direction and our lives with a sense.

Contrary to our dominant presumptions, we are seldom conscious of what we are doing or who we are. We choose to stay ignorant of certain engagements with the world, for to put them all together often asks too much of us, and sometimes threatens the more enjoyable engagements. We profess sincerity and normally try to abide by that profession, yet we neglect to acquire the very skills which will test that profession of sincerity against our current performance. On the contrary, we deliberately allow certain engagements to go unexamined, quite aware that areas left unaccountable tend to cater to self-interest. As a result of that inertial policy, the condition of self-deception becomes the rule rather than the exception in our lives, and often in the measure that we are trying to be honest and sincere. Sobering as this fact is, however, it does not license a wholesale charge of hypocrisy. Self-deception remains more subtle.

Some of our self-deceptions, moreover, have more destructive results than others. Auschwitz stands as a symbol of one extreme to which our self-deception can lead. For the complicity of Christians with Auschwitz did not begin with their failure to object to the first slightly anti-Semitic laws and actions. It rather began when Christians assumed that they could be the heirs and carriers of the symbols of the faith without sacrifice and suffering. It began when the very language of revelation became an expression of status rather than an instrument for bringing our lives gradually under the sway of "the love that moves the sun and the other stars." Persons had come to call themselves Christians and yet live as though they could avoid suffering and death. So Christians allowed their language to idle without turning the engines of the soul, and in recompense, their lives were seized by powers that they no longer had the ability to know, much less to combat.

It is not likely that anyone reading this actually cooperated with Auschwitz, but the conditions of self-deception that created Auschwitz still prevail in our souls. We prefer to believe that the powers of darkness that reigned at Auschwitz have left the scent of combat, overcome by the sheer horror of what happened there. But we cannot afford to ignore Auschwitz, for to overlook it sets the stage for yet further self-deception. Moreover, by forgetting Auschwitz we neglect the grammar of the language we have learned from the cross of Christ.

This essay is divided into three sections: the first offers a preliminary philosophical analysis of self-deception; the second examines Speer's claim of self-deception in *Inside the Third Reich;* the third attempts to delineate some conditions necessary to live our lives more truthfully. The specific convictions about ethical life and reflection which shape this essay are not made explicit here. We cannot do better, however, as a way of summarizing the general position than to endorse David Harned's claim that:

> Seeing is never simply a reaction to what passes before our eyes; it is a matter of how well the eye is trained and provisioned to discern the richness and the terror, beauty and banality of the worlds outside and within the self. Decisions are shaped by vision, and the ways that we see are a function of our "character," of the history and habits of the self, and ultimately of the stories that we have heard and with which we identify ourselves. More precisely seeing is determined by the constellation of images of man and the world that resides within the household of the self. Sometimes they inhibit and corrupt a person as much as they sustain him, but their common source is always faith, the tangle of loyalties that the self has developed in the course of time. . . . The real problem, however, is not the variety of faiths we entertain or images of man by which we are all beset, not their partiality, nor even the conflicts among them, but our need for a master image of the self that can reconcile the lesser ones that draw a person first one way

and then another toward conflicting goals, each of them claiming greater authority than it deserves, promising greater rewards than it can provide.[1]

This essay is an attempt to illustrate these claims by showing the inadequacy of one man's master image. While we write as Christians and believe that Speer's case bears peculiarly upon Christians, we do not believe our analysis and reflections are confined in their import to Christians.

2.   Self-Deception: A Theoretical Account

As familiar as we are with self-deception, we find it elusive to get hold of analytically. We tend to think of self-deception as a case of self-lying, but lying to oneself turns out to be a paradoxical enterprise. A mother may maintain that her son is a good boy when all the evidence indicates he is not, but we assume that she really knows differently. Confidence in her son may be a strategy to straighten him out by creating certain expectations or an attempt to ward off the shame she thinks she should feel for rearing such a son. Many other explanations could be offered for her state of self-deception, but explanations of this type all conspire to deny that the mother is genuinely self-deceived. She would not be deceived if she merely told herself that he was a good boy; she must be convinced that he is.

Self-deception must stem from a purpose strong enough that our position cannot be interpreted as a sham. The model of self-lying overlooks intentional or purposive origins of self-deception and leaves us in a paradoxical situation. To be sure, self-deception often seems to involve the co-existence in one person of two incompatible beliefs, but when individual cases are so analyzed they turn out to be something other than self-deception. For the agent must be assumed to be aware of both beliefs while playing like he or she does not hold one of them. We know, however, that we do not just play at self-deception. For we have often come to realize how deceived we have been, yet quite unsuspectingly all the while.

2.1   Consciousness as Knowing How

Our rudimentary view of consciousness as awareness will not suffice to offer a plausible account of self-deception. We presume that we are conscious of our activity since we seem to be aware of what we are doing most of the time. But this is hardly the case. I can be conscious of what I am doing without perceiving myself doing it, and I can be aware of what I am up to yet fail to take it into account. Furthermore, to think of being conscious as "taking a look" is not only misleading but leads to an analytical regress, since every intentional act (including looking) is deemed to be conscious.[2] Consciousness is more like an ability to say than the power to see. Our native powers of consciousness are susceptible of progressive training. It would not be amiss to insist that we must be trained to be conscious.

Herbert Fingarette offers the model of an operating skill to replace the more passive image of awareness, and shows how the skill-model can elaborate our sense of being explicitly conscious.

> To become explicitly conscious of something is to be exercising a certain skill. Skills, of course, are learned but need not be routinized. We are born with certain general capacities which we shape, by learning, into specific skills, some of them being quite sensitive and artful. The specific skill I particularly have in mind as a model for becoming explicitly conscious of something is the skill of saying what we are doing or experiencing. I propose, then, that we do not characterize consciousness as a kind of mental mirror, but as the exercise of the (learned) skill of 'spelling out' some feature of the world we are engaged in.[3]

To become explicitly conscious of one's situation, then, demands that one rehearse what one is doing. We seldom feel it necessary to spell out our engagements in any detail, however. Conventional descriptions of our actions are readily available, and they normally dispense us from spelling things out any further. There are many things we do every day—dressing, eating, playing with our children or talking with our spouses—that can be carried on without bothering to delineate how they may contribute to an overall life-plan. We seldom "spell out" what we are doing unless we are prodded to do so: "Rather than taking explicit consciousness for granted; we must see explicit consciousness as the further exercise of a specific skill for special reasons."[4]

Furthermore, at times we sense it to be a more reasonable policy *not* to spell out some of our engagements. By adopting such a policy, however, we not only avoid becoming explicitly conscious. We also set up a situation that allows us to avoid becoming explicitly conscious that we are avoiding it. It is this very reduplication, of course, that insures self-deception. By suggesting that we regard explicit consciousness as perfecting a native ability to spell things out, Fingarette renders the curiously reflexive maneuver a bit more plausible. The mother who insists her son is good when he is engaged in doubtful activities not only refuses to apply her ordinary criteria for right and wrong in this case. She also avoids recognizing that she is not employing these criteria as she normally does. To bring certain things to consciousness requires the moral stamina to endure the pain that such explicit knowledge cannot help but bring. The mother's self-deception plays a supportive role by staving off the pain that would inevitably accompany her spelling out what her son's behavior entails.

2.2   An Avoidance Policy

We can now offer a preliminary account of what self-deception involves. A self-deceived person is one of whom "it is a patent characteristic that even when normally appropriate he *persistently* avoids spelling out some feature of his engagement with the world."[5] A state of self-deception cannot issue from a single decision, then, but represents a policy not to spell out certain activities in which the agent is involved. Moreover, once such a policy has been adopted, there is ever more reason to continue it, so that a process of self-deception has been initiated. Our overall posture of sincerity demands that we make this particular policy consistent with the whole range of our engagements. In this way, a specific policy leads to a pervasive condition called self-deception. Curiously enough, it is our prevailing desire to be consistent which escalates a policy into an enveloping condition. Thus the mother in our example may begin to believe that there is a conspiracy by school and correctional officials to discredit her son. Our protective deceits become destructive when they begin to serve our need to shape a world consistent with our illusions. The power of fabrication makes it that much harder to uncover our deceptions by masking them with sufficient plausibility to render them acceptable. Occasionally we are fortunate enough to be forced to face our deceptions, but ironically the very same imaginative and intellectual skills which lead us to discriminate falsity from truth also empower us to create those webs of illusion that lend plausibility to our original deceptive policy.

We may even feel that the commitments we have made require us to keep up an ongoing policy of avoidance. We may feel compelled to maintain our web of illusion because we have drawn others into it. We can quiet any misgivings we may have for fear of the injury which spelling things out could inflict upon those who love us. Jules Henry's *Pathways in Madness*,[6] an account of families of psychotic children, offers a tragic commentary on the avoidance strategies some families have elaborated, ostensibly to preserve the love they have achieved. It so happens, however, that one of their members must pay the toll for a policy that tries to preserve a love story by overlooking certain disharmonious subplots.

Our lives are replete with illusions for they constitute an essential part of our coping equipment. Henry points out how professors can continue to act as if they were effective teachers when they are not, because they must feel effective to earn a living to support their family. There are often moral reasons to sustain the illusions of our lives. Consider the many conversations with others that appear to be congenial but which may bore or otherwise annoy both parties, "yet each person harbors the necessary illusion that he is pulling the wool over the other person's eyes. The illusions must be maintained in order for people to carry on. The illusion of concealment, of safety, of deceiving the other are part of the absolutely necessary structure of consciousness. The illusion keeps us sane."[7]

The complexity and extent of our self-deception explains why we avoid spelling out our engagements. Each of us needs to establish some sense of identity and unity in order to give coherence to the multifariousness of our history as uniquely ours and as constitutive of the self.[8] Self-deception can accompany this need for unity, as we systematically delude ourselves in order to maintain the story that has hitherto assured our identity. We hesitate to spell out certain engagements when spelling them out would jeopardize the set of avowals we have made about ourselves.

Societal roles provide a ready vehicle for self-deception, since we can easily identify with them without any need to spell out what we are doing. The role is accepted into our identity. It may define our identity in the measure that we feel committed to live out and defend our identification with it. In the narrow confines of a job and of corporate loyalty, such an individual can easily be caricatured as a "company man," and come under a simple censure of establishment myopia. Where the description is more exalted and vocational, however, the opportunity for deceiving oneself increases. A man may think of himself as a public servant concerned with the public good. Even though he may be party to decisions which compromise the public good, he has a great deal invested in continuing to describe them as contributing to the public good. To call certain decisions he makes by their proper name would require too painful a readjustment in his primary identification of himself as a public servant. Thus our deceit can be a function of wanting to think of ourselves as honest persons.

The irony of self-deception is that a cynic is less vulnerable to self-deception than a conscientious person.

> The less integrity, the less is there motive to enter into self-deception. The greater the integrity of the person, and the more powerful the contrary inclination, the greater is the temptation to self-deception (the nearer to saintliness, the more a powerful personality suffers). It is because the movement into self-deception is rooted in a concern for integrity of spirit that we temper our condemnation of the self-deceiver. We feel he is not a *mere* cheat. We are moved to a certain comparison in which there is awareness of the self-deceiver's authentic inner dignity as the motive of his self-betrayal.[9]

What the self-deceiver lacks is not integrity or sincerity but the courage and skill to confront the reality of his or her situation. Self-deception is correlative with trying to exist in this life without a story sufficiently substantive and rich to sustain us in the unavoidable challenges that confront the self. It may be possible to "function effectively" without such a story, but to do so we necessarily reduce our rightful expectations and interests. To live bravely is to be willing to risk our present lives in pursuing the consequences of the commitments we have made. A policy of fidelity cannot help but challenge the story we currently hold about ourselves. We can afford to let go of our current story, however, only to the extent that we are convinced that it does not hold the key to our individual identity. So we will remain subject to those propensities which lead to a state of self-deception as long as we feel ourself to be constituted either by the conventional roles we have assumed or by the level of awareness we have been able to articulate. Alternatively, we will have some leverage on these powers in the measure that we believe ourself to be constituted by a story given to us by a power beyond our will or imagination.

2.3 Discriminating Stories

In summary, self-deception results from an expedient policy of refusing to spell out our engagements in order to preserve the particular identity we have achieved. The extent of our self-deception correlates with the type of story we hold about who and what we are. If it is to counter our propensity to self-deception, the story that sustains our life must give us the ability to spell out in advance the limits of the various roles we will undertake in our lives. The story must enable us to discriminate within those roles the behavior that can easily entrap and blind us. The more noble and caring the role, the more discriminating the story must be. To lack such a story, as we shall see in the case of Speer, is to be deprived of the skills necessary to recognize or challenge the demonic. And to be bereft of those skills is to fall prey to these powers. That much we can now say, after Auschwitz.

3. Albert Speer: The Life of an Architect

Speer's autobiography can be read as one long confession of self-deception. As he says of himself, "I have always thought it was a most valuable trait to recognize reality and not to pursue delusions. But when I now think over my life up to and including the years of imprisonment, there was no period in which I was free of delusory notions."[10] Rather than try to use his self-deceit as an excuse for participation in Hitler's government, Speer explicitly states that he accepts and should accept full responsibility for all the crimes committed by Hitler—including the murder of six million Jews.

We cannot help but ask, however, whether Speer's admission is not an extremely clever way of reclaiming his place in decent society. For is not claiming responsibility for the murder of the Jews an empty gesture? What could anyone do to render such a claim credible? Even the theme of self-deception seems to give Speer a kind of legitimacy and integrity that excuses his active participation in Hitler's government. How are we to connect, in other words, the admissions of the autobiography with the life Speer led as a Nazi?[11]

3.1 The Account

Speer's account rings true. He recognizes how impossible it is to claim responsibility for the murder of the Jews. Only when we again see the pictures of the bodies and the ovens filled with bones can we even begin to imagine that reign of death. It is not the murder of the six million that we comprehend, but the murder of the one person or family that we see in a picture. Speer does not claim to see all six million but says he is haunted by the "account of a Jewish family going to their deaths: the husband with his wife and children on the way to die are before my eyes to this day" (Speer, p. 25). It is less agonizing to claim responsibility for the murder of six million as their very number makes them an abstraction, but Speer recognizes that such a claim means that he helped murder this family.

Speer's account of his activities as a Nazi is corroborated by other investigation. Trevor-Roper criticizes Speer severely, but acknowledges that his conclusions about the war and his involvement in it

> are never naive, never parochial; they seem always honest; they are often profound. If he seems sometimes to have fallen too deeply under the spell of the tyrant whom he served, at least he is the only servant whose judgment was not corrupted by attendance on that dreadful master; at least he retained the capacity to examine himself, and the honesty to declare both his errors and his convictions. In the last days of Nazism he was not afraid to tell Hitler of his own acts of defiance; and in Allied captivity he was not afraid to admit, after his searching analysis of Hitler's character and history, the residue of loyalty which he could not altogether shed.[12]

Ironically enough, testimonies like these to Speer's personal integrity undermine our trust in his account. For we fail to see how a man of integrity and substance could have served Hitler so well. What staggers us is not what Arendt in describing Eichmann called the banality of evil, but the reality of a good man serving such masters.[13] It would be easier if we could think of Speer as a dedicated and committed Nazi, for then his actions would be intelligible. Perhaps Speer's confession of self-deception carries us beyond an attempt to

clear his own name. He is reminding us that integrity and sincerity in themselves are not sufficient safeguards against the seduction of evil.[14]

But how could a man like Speer become involved in so monstrous a self-
deception? He was a man who could make realistic assessments. He was
among the first to realize that the war could not be won because Allied
bombing made it impossible for Germany to match the Allies' technological
capacity (Speer, p. 445). He was also a keen observer of the faults and
pettiness of the men around Hitler. Notwithstanding his strong personal at-
tachment to Hitler, Speer almost singlehandedly, and with great courage,
stayed the execution of Hitler's scorched-earth policy against Germany (Speer,
p. 565).[15]

Nothing in Speer's background would seem to have led him into the company of Nazis. He came from a prosperous and professional family and he
enjoyed a happy childhood. Even though politics was seldom discussed at
home, his father was a liberal committed to social reform. Speer received an
excellent education and admits himself that as an intellectual he should have
been repulsed by Hitler's crude propaganda. That aspect of Nazism he simply
ignored, however, as politics and not to be taken seriously (Speer, p. 48). At
his father's urging he continued the family tradition by becoming an architect,
studying under one of the finest architects in Germany, and even becoming his
assistant. He fell in love, married, and seems to have been a humane and
loving father.

Yet this same man served as Hitler's Minister of Armaments. Many esti-
mate his accomplishments lengthened the war by at least two years. For some
time Speer was the second most powerful man in Germany as he organized
Germany's industry to provide the military hardware for Hitler's armies. In
that capacity he also approved of and willingly accepted the use of slave labor
in Germany's factories and mines. It was this policy that earned him twenty
years in prison at Nuremberg.

He not only knew slave labor was being used; he saw the inhumane conditions under which these men lived and worked. He did try to assure them at
least minimal living conditions, but he was forced to admit that he really did
not see these men at all.

> What preys on my mind nowadays has little to do with the standards of
> Nuremberg nor the figures on lives I saved or might have saved. For in
> either case I was moving within the system. What disturbs me more is that I
> failed to read the physiognomy of the regime mirrored in the faces of those
> prisoners—the regime whose existence I was so obsessively trying to pro-
> long during those weeks and months. I did not see any moral ground
> outside the system where I should have taken my stand. And sometimes I
> ask myself who this young man really was, this young man who has now
> become so alien to me, who walked through the workshops of the Linz

steelworks or descended into the caverns of the Central Works twenty-five years ago (Speer, p. 480).

Even though Speer never thought of himself as anti-Semitic and took no part in the destruction of the Jews, he also admits that he deliberately made himself blind to what was happening to the Jews. Because he felt no hatred toward the Jews, he assumed that he had no involvement in their harassment. He saw the burned-out synagogues but reacted quite indifferently. For as he says, "I felt myself to be Hitler's architect. Political events did not concern me" (Speer, p. 162). Later he was warned by his friend, Gauleiter Karl Hanke, never to go to Auschwitz. Speer admits he purposely refused to ask him why. Nor did he ask Himmler or Hitler or anyone else from whom he could have easily found out the truth.

> For I did not want to know what was happening there. During those few seconds, while Hanke was warning me, the whole responsibility had become a reality again. Those seconds were uppermost in my mind when I stated to the international court at the Nuremberg Trial that as an important member of the leadership of the Reich, I had to share the total responsibility for all that had happened. For from that moment on, I was inescapably contaminated morally; from fear of discovering something which might have made me turn from my course. I had closed my eyes. This deliberate blindness outweighs whatever good I may have done or tried to do in the last period of the war. Those activities shrink to nothing in the face of it. Because I failed at that time, I still feel to this day responsible for Auschwitz in the wholly personal sense (Speer, p. 481).

3.2 His Story

But how did Speer get to the point that there was "no moral ground outside the system"? Why would any man make himself "deliberately blind"? Speer knew that the knowledge of Auschwitz—if articulated—would destroy his very being. He had no skill to explain such a horror and still know how to go on as the young man he had become. His original commitment to Hitler offered him a ready reason for refusing to spell out the consequences of his present involvements. His self-deception was correlative to his identity as he clung to the story of being Hitler's apolitical architect. As Speer says, "my new political interests played a subsidiary part in my thinking. I was above all an architect" (Speer, p. 51).[16]

But he was an architect born and trained in a defeated country. He aspired to erect monuments to the human spirit, but he lived in a country ready only to build garages. Hitler offered Speer hope; he offered him a vision, a story of a country which would again ask its architects to raise up public buildings.

What Hitler offered Speer is what every professional dreams of, the opportunity to make his wildest ambitions come true. The long chapters describing the architectural plans he worked on with Hitler display the extent of these ambitions.

Speer cared nothing for politics in itself. He thought National Socialism was a better alternative than communism, but such considerations were not what led him to join the party. He joined the party and was increasingly drawn into its activities because, as he says, "My position as Hitler's architect had soon become indispensable to me. Not yet thirty, I saw before me the most exciting prospects an architect can dream of" (Speer, p. 64).

Hitler gave Speer the opportunity to lose himself in his work: assured identity with the equal security of serving a high ideal. Everything else would have to give way, of course, and Speer gave up "the real center of my life: my family. Completely under the sway of Hitler, I was henceforth possessed by my work" (Speer, p. 64). As one architectural assignment followed another, Speer had less and less reason to spell out the engagement he had begun. He knew what he was doing: he was an architect. No more was needed.

Even when he became Minister of Armaments Speer continued to think of himself primarily as an architect. The reorganization of German industry to serve the ends of war was a creative technological task with which he could readily identify. This new position was a natural extension of the skills learned from his architectural training; he brought form in a different medium through technological manipulation. In this highly political task he could continue to disdain politics as perverting the ends of efficiency and good order. So Speer's new position did not require him to rethink the master image of his life: he continued to be above all an architect.

What he failed to appreciate, of course, was how seductive and destructive it was to be "Hitler's architect" (Speer, p. 64). Seductive because it put him on intimate terms with power, as the picture he draws of himself arriving for lunch at his new chancellery betrays so candidly: "The policeman at the entrance to the front garden knew my car and opened the gate without making inquiries. . . . The SS member of Hitler's escort squad greeted me familiarly" (Speer, p. 168). Destructive even of his architectural sense, as a chance auto trip through Castile in 1941 warned him. Remarking on the Escorial of Philip II, he recaptures his sentiments at that time: "What a contrast with Hitler's architectural ideas: in the one case, remarkable conciseness and clarity, magnificent interior rooms, their forms perfectly controlled; in the other case, pomp and disproportionate ostentation. . . . In hours of solitary contemplation it began to dawn on me for the first time that my recent architectural ideals were on the wrong track" (Speer, p. 251). Yet the insight proved inoperable. The architect in him had become Hitler's architect.

It was later when he began to write his autobiography that Speer realized how "before 1944 I so rarely—in fact almost never—found the time to reflect about myself or my own activities, that I never gave my own existence a thought. Today, in retrospect, I often have the feeling that something swept me up off the ground at the time, wrenched me from all roots, and beamed a host of alien forces upon me" (Speer, p. 64). Towards the end of the war Speer was able to distance himself from Hitler's will to realize that the future of Germany overreached that of Hitler (Speer, p. 574). Yet that very patriotism had drawn him to Hitler originally. He had no effective way to step back from himself, no place to stand. His self-deception began when he assumed that "being above all an architect" was a story sufficient to constitute his self. He had to experience the solitude of prison to realize that becoming a human being requires stories and images a good deal richer than professional ones, if we are to be equipped to deal with the powers of this world.

3.3 The Lesson Presented

As a justification for writing his story Speer says he intends the book to be a warning to the future (Speer, p. 659). But it is not clear exactly what that warning is. A ready candidate for "a lesson for the future" seems to be Speer's final speech at Nuremberg as he warned of the potential tyrannical use of technology:

> Hitler's dictatorship was the first dictatorship of an industrial state in this age of modern technology. A dictatorship which employed to perfection the instruments of technology to dominate its own people. . . . Dictatorship of the past needed assistants of high quality in the lower ranks of the leadership also—men who could think and act independently. The authoritarian system in the age of technology can do without such men. The means of communication alone enable it to mechanize the work of the lower leadership. Thus the type of uncritical receiver of orders is created (Speer, p. 654).

We suspect, however, that the warning lies closer to Speer's own life than his direct remarks can say. The British newspaper article from *The Observer* (April 9, 1944) that Speer showed Hitler to prevent Bormann from using it against him is closer to the truth. It suggested that even though Speer was not one of the flamboyant and picturesque Nazis, he was more important to Germany than Hitler, Himmler, Goering, or the generals. For Speer

> is very much the successful average man, well-dressed, civil, noncorrupt, very middle class in his style of life, with a wife and six children. Much less

than any of the other German leaders does he stand for anything particularly German or particularly Nazi. He rather symbolizes a type which is becoming increasingly important in all belligerent countries: the pure technician, the classless bright young man without background, with no other original aim than to make his way in the world and no other means than his technical and managerial ability. It is the lack of psychological and spiritual ballast, and the ease with which he handles the terrifying technical and organizational machinery of our age, which makes this slight type go extremely far nowadays. . . . This is their age; the Hitlers, the Himmlers we may get rid of, but the Speers, whatever happens to this particular special man, will long be with us (Speer, p. 443).

Speer's reflections reach beyond the potential dangers of technology to warn us about people who think they need no story or skills beyond their profession. Such people are open to manipulation by anyone who offers them a compelling vision of how that skill can be used. We all require a sense of worth, a sense of place in the human enterprise, and the person with no story beyond his or her role yearns to be so placed by another. We yearn for a cause in which we can lose ourselves. Persons with no politics become political pawns, lacking as they do the skills to grasp the shape of their involvements.

Speer was a man who began his engagement with life with a story inadequate to articulate the engagements he would be called upon to undertake. He shared the German distrust of things political and turned instead to his profession, where he had the satisfaction (along with the illusion) of "knowing what he was doing." Trevor-Roper argues that from this perspective Speer is the most culpable of the Nazis. For

it is quite clear that in Hitler's court Albert Speer was morally and intellectually alone. He had the capacity to understand the forces of politics, and the courage to resist the master whom all others have declared irresistible. As an administrator, he was undoubtedly a genius. He regarded the rest of the court with dignified contempt. His ambitions were peaceful and constructive: he wished to rebuild Berlin and Nuremberg, and had planned to make them the greatest cities in the world. Nevertheless, in a political sense, Speer is the real criminal of Nazi Germany, for he more than any other, represented the fatal philosophy which has made havoc of Germany and nearly shipwrecked the world. For ten years he sat at the very center of political power; his keen intelligence diagnosed the nature, and observed the mutations of Nazi government and policy; he saw and despised personalities around him; he heard the outrageous orders and understood their fantastic ambitions; but he did nothing. Supposing politics to be irrelevant, he turned aside, and built roads and bridges and factories, while the logical consequences of government by madmen emerged. Ultimately, when their emergence involved the ruin of all his work, Speer accepted the consequences and acted. Then it was too late; Germany had been destroyed.[17]

Speer's life warns us, certainly, of possible misuses of technology, but the warning is directed more accurately against those who feel they need no images and symbols beyond those offered by conventional roles to give coherence to their lives. We have thought that the way to drive out the evil gods was to deny the existence of all gods. In fact, however, we have found ourselves serving a false god that is all the more powerful because we fail to recognize it as a god.[18] Yet the gods, it seems, will have their due. Any story which overlooks the powers must pretend that the self can be constituted by the roles one has assumed or by the current story a person has been able to compose. Yet neither of these will suffice, as we have seen, for each of them is susceptible of confirming us in a state of self-deception.

A true story could only be one powerful enough to check the endemic tendency toward self-deception—a tendency which inadequate stories cannot help but foster. Correlatively, if the true God were to provide us with a saving story, it would have to be one that we found continually discomforting. For it would be a saving story only as it empowered us to combat the inertial drift into self-deception.

4. Story, Skill and the Knowledge of Evil

To be is to be rooted in self-deception. The moral task involves a constant vigilance: to note those areas where the tendency has taken root. This task is made more difficult by the illusions of the past which we have unsuspectingly inherited. Even the wisdom of the last generation fails to serve us as it did our fathers, since we have received it without a struggle. Principles, too, that have served to guide one part of our lives can countenance destructive activity if we unwittingly press them into service in other areas. Love of country that once inspired noble deeds can lead us to commit the worst crimes when we have lost the skills to recognize how other loyalties must qualify that of patriotism.

Rather than demand whether it was possible to avoid self-deception, we should rather try to assess how effectively deceived we have become. Our ability to "step-back"[19] from our deceptions is dependent on the dominant story, the master image, that we have embodied in our character.[20] Through our experience we constantly learn new lessons, we gain new insights, about the limit of our life story. But "insights are a dime a dozen"[21] and even more useless unless we have the skills—the images and the stories—which can empower those insights to shape our lives. It is not enough to see nor is it enough to know; we must know how to say and give expression to what we come to see and know. "Understanding what something is demands more than insight or vision—it requires appropriate discipline."[22]

Like Columbus, we all have encounters that we do not know how to describe. Our basic stories and images determine what we discover, but often, like Columbus, we insist on describing our engagements with an image that misleads us. To the extent that we cannot make anything of what we are doing, we fail to make our lives into anything. Columbus could not understand what he had done because he did not have the skills to get it right. Fortunately, we can keep sending out our ships to explore the coastlines of our engagements and learn the limits of our past descriptions; and on the strength of previous failures, we can develop more adequate skills to say what we have done. Too often, however, we adopt the first coherent description of what we have done and it leads to greater self-deception. Our endemic need for order—the same demand we experience to make a story of our lives—also presses us to forge a unity before we have discovered one adequate to our situation. Hence the inertial tendency to a state of self-deception.

4.1   Art of Articulation

The art of autobiography offers the best illustration of how to recheck and test the adequacy of the central story and image we have of our lives. The constraints and requirements of autobiography parallel those of a life well-lived. Like the moral person, the autobiographer cannot simply recount the events of his or her life. He or she must write from the dominant perspective and image of his or her present time. If this effort is successful, these images and metaphors will provide the skills to articulate the limits of past images and show how they have led to the autobiographer's current perspective. Autobiography is the literary form that mirrors the moral necessity to free ourselves from the hold of our illusions by exercising the skills which more demanding stories provide. Autobiography is the literary act that rehearses our liberation from illusory goals by showing how to bring specific skills of understanding to bear on our desires and aversions, so that an intelligible pattern emerges. An autobiographer, like a moral person, needs to find a story that gives a life coherence without distorting the quality of his or her actual engagements with others and with the world.

This requirement means that skill cannot be confused with technique, for the skills required to ferret out the truth cannot be separated from the images that sustain the skill. We need a story that allows us to recognize the evil we do and enables us to accept responsibility for it in a non-destructive way. We sense far too accurately the suffering that the knowledge of evil can cause, and we comfort ourselves with deceptions that excuse. We live out stories that attempt to free us from the terrible knowledge that our sins are real. We fear such knowledge because we sense how it can destroy whatever we have managed to become and paralyze our ability to act. How can we know the truth about ourselves and still know how to go on?

Malcolm X came to realize that he could not avoid becoming a "white man's nigger." Yet he could hardly afford to admit the self-hate symbolized by straightening his hair, for such knowledge would have destroyed him completely. Instead, he swallowed his dignity and survived by learning the small hustles that white men allowed blacks to perpetrate on one another. There was no story readily available that could give him the skill to recognize the truth about himself without destroying everything. For how do you recognize that you have been a "white man's nigger" and know how to go on?

The story of the Black Muslims that Malcolm learned in prison provided the precise skill necessary for him to face up to his situation.[23] The story offered an explanation of why blacks in America necessarily became the "white man's nigger," and that interpretation gave him the skills to know how to go on. This story intended to create a new people, to prepare for a new exodus, in effect to bestow a new name. The story also gave institutional skills which could be embodied in ritual and gestures: cease eating pork, participate in the temple and accept the disciplined life that frees from the white man's ways and stereotypes. Any story that fails to provide institutional forms is power-less, for it is not enough merely to offer the story. One must know how to tell it in such a way that persons can become the story.

Malcolm's story cannot be ours, however—if we are white, Christian and American or even European—for the evil he had to recognize is not the same as ours. Malcolm had to learn to live as the victim and the ravaged; we must learn to live as the victor and the ravager. For we are people who not only have the suppression of the blacks to our name, but the reality of Auschwitz as part of our history. Like slavery, Auschwitz was not an accidental sideshow to the main events of Western Christendom. We cannot ask the Jew, any more than we can ask the black, to forget that these things have been done by Christians. No reconciliation is possible between white and black, Jew and Christian, unless we can learn to carry the burden of these past crimes.

5. Concluding Reflections

Our problem is not unlike Speer's, for we too must find a place and perspective from which we can write our story without distortion. We must learn how to hold the guilt that such a story brings without trying to rid ourselves of it by morbid self-denunciation or false gestures of identifying with our victim. Speer reveals little of the perspective from which he now writes his life. Perhaps he is wise enough to know that his past deceptions would make any explicit statement of his current convictions problematic. Whatever wisdom he has gained is better shown than said. Beyond that, silence would appear a more truthful policy.

But wisdom needs more than silence, for understanding comes only through images. Christians claim to find the skill to confess the evil that we do in the history of Jesus Christ.[24] It is a history of suffering and death that must be made our own if we are to mine its significance. The saints formed by this story testify to its efficacy in purging the self of all deception as it forces the acceptance of a new self mirrored in the cross. Moreover, this story has given the saints a way to go on as they become disciples of the way—the way of learning to deal with evil without paying back in kind.

The stories that produce truthful lives are those that provide the skills to step back and survey the limits of our engagements. Nations, no less than individuals, require such stories. These stories will help us to recognize and acknowledge the evil we perpetrate and to confront ourselves without illusion and deceit. Our urge to be good, to have a coherent and unified self, and our need to have a sense of worth are strong. We will do almost anything to avoid recognizing the limits on our claims to righteousness.[25] In fact, we seem to be able to acknowledge those limits only when life has brought us to the point where we can do nothing else. To accept the Gospel is to receive training in accepting the limits on our claims to righteousness before we are forced to. It is a hard and painful discipline but it cannot be avoided, we suspect, if we wish to have a place to stand free of self-deception.

PART TWO

Survival, Community
and the Demand for Truthfulness

6. Memory, Community
and the Reasons for Living:
Reflections on Suicide and Euthanasia

with Richard Bondi

> If suicide is allowed then everything is allowed. If anything is not
> allowed then suicide is not allowed. This throws a light on the nature of
> ethics, for suicide is, so to speak, the elementary sin.
>
> Wittgenstein, *Notebooks,* 1914–1925

1. Suicide and Euthanasia as Moral Problems

Ethicists do not need to provide a reason to describe suicide and euthanasia
as moral problems. Everyone seems to agree that if anything is a moral
problem suicide and euthanasia are prime examples and thus ready grist for the
ethicist's mill. As Wittgenstein suggests, we seem to be on fundamentally
moral grounds when dealing with the taking of one's own life.

Yet we feel it is by no means clear why it is assumed that suicide and
euthanasia raise moral issues, or indeed, what those issues are and how the
ethicist might relate to them. At the very least people have begun to realize
that "acts" of suicide and euthanasia are often ambiguous. We suspect,
however, that the unanimous agreement that suicide and euthanasia constitute
moral problems is not connected with such practical cases. Rather it reflects
an increasingly prevalent judgement that the traditional assumption that
suicide and euthanasia are morally questionable has itself become problematic.[1] Some are suggesting that suicide and euthanasia are not only morally
ambiguous, but that they represent positive moral goods or rights. This is
particularly true in relation to euthanasia, which often appears a kind and
humane act.[2] Thus while the place of suicide and euthanasia on a list of
"moral problems" is still secure, how the notions are to be understood is no
longer clear.

We do not believe that the way out of this difficulty lies in constructing ever more comprehensive typologies of suicide and euthanasia. Rather we must try to get at the grammar of the notions. In this essay we will examine 'suicide' and 'euthanasia' as heuristic notions to see how they may be displayed in a given community. We are specifically interested in how these notions relate to the story that forms the Christian community. Indeed, we will suggest that the notions of suicide and euthanasia are incompatible with and subversive of some fundamental elements of the Christian story. At the same time our investigation should have wider appeal. Our attempt represents a model of how the moral notions and practical behavior of any people relate to the story that constitutes it as community. In this way we also hope to open up the possibility for challenges to the Christian tradition being made intelligible themselves in terms of the use of moral notions within a story that they embody.

1.1   The Ambiguity of Suicide and Euthanasia as Moral Notions

If this is true, it should make us wary of the "hard case" approach, which proceeds by examining certain instances of actual or potential suicide or euthanasia.[3] The assumption is that we already know what euthanasia or suicide is and the task is to find counter-examples that will let you ask what is wrong with suicide or euthanasia under X or Y circumstances. We are suggesting instead that the ambiguity is in the notions of suicide and euthanasia themselves, and more particularly in the role they play in relation to the story that shapes our moral vocabulary.

The hard case approach, with its emphasis on discrete acts, is backwards, as it assumes that the moral life is primarily concerned with decisions. Yet prior to the question of "what should we do" is the question "what should we be." For "what we are" is the context that makes moral notions such as suicide and euthanasia work at all. Suicide and euthanasia are not just descriptions of individual acts, but notions that form intentionality to have one kind of character rather than another. It is this latter kind of problem that is our concern in this essay, namely, not what we should do in certain contexts, but what kind of character we should have in order to see certain contexts one way rather than another. Or even more accurately we are concerned with what kind of communities we should be to encourage people to view their death as a humane ending that we need not hasten through our own power. We are concerned with what kind of story a community needs to hold about life that provides the skills to display the notions of suicide and euthanasia in a morally accurate way. Put differently, when the moral question is limited to whether certain assumed acts are suicide or euthanasia, and thus to be praised or blamed, we often fail to see the positive commitments embodied in such notions. Suicide and euthanasia as notions that help individuate certain behavior involve background beliefs without which their descriptive value is limited or perhaps misleading.[4]

This can be illustrated by considering what we mean by suicide. "The taking of one's own life" is clearly insufficient. We would not wish to admit to a moral vocabulary so impoverished as to lump together Saul or those who died at Massada with the student who plunges from an eighth-story window after failing to make fraternity rush. Yet if we begin to make distinctions we must ultimately appeal, not to the physical description of the act, but to the meaning it has in the larger social, moral and cultural context. In other words, we are back to examining the formal notions of suicide and euthanasia in relation to the stories which shape our communities. As Jack Douglas has pointed out, the social meaning of suicide is in part constructed by the person committing the act, but is fundamentally in the hands of the community where the formation of the moral notions and vocabulary which the suicide uses in "constructing" his or her act takes place.[5]

We may assume that euthanasia is easier to describe than suicide since it seems to be a more limited case. That this is not the case can be seen in the contrast between the etymology of the word and its present usage. The word originally meant simply "good death."[6] However, it currently means the ending of life in order to secure the release from pain and suffering; or more rigorously put, it is the deliberate, intended putting to death of someone in pain in order to secure their release from pain. It is obvious that this description attempts to qualify some acts of putting ourselves or someone to death from all the material acts of death that involve release from pain. In other words, not all cases that look like euthanasia carry the moral weight normally associated with the judgment implied in the notion of euthanasia.[7] In the case of both suicide and euthanasia, only an examination of the stories that form the notions can help us understand and use them properly.[8]

1.2 The Importance of Attitudes toward Life-taking

It is impossible to understand suicide or euthanasia apart from our attitudes toward life itself. We should not view these issues as special cases of death but as the result of certain attitudes toward life. It is this that ties the two issues together—if we learn to think morally about suicide in terms of our willingness to live we will have gained the necessary skills to talk about euthanasia.

When an ethicist takes on issues such as euthanasia or suicide, it looks like his or her primary interest is to tell us whether a particular set of actions are right or wrong, to be encouraged or discouraged. But rather our job is to help the communities we serve to keep their language pure—in other words, the ethicist is more like a poet than anything else. Our primary interest in this essay is to help Christians get the meaning of suicide and euthanasia right in terms of how those notions help them to understand the basic story that defines the kind of community they are.

Thus, identifying the grammar of suicide and euthanasia entails discriminating the story that the notions play a role in. Our notions, our descriptions, our very actions are held fast by stories, by the narratives which are our context for meaning.[9] Ethics is the attempt to help us remember what kind of story sustains certain descriptions. It is, therefore, a discipline rather like history, in that we are forced to tell stories in order to capture our past, sustain our present, and give our future direction.[10]

It may be that the meaning of suicide and euthanasia for Christians is the same as that found in our wider society, but that is certainly not self-evident. As Christian ethicists, we may well share a story that you do not, though we hope that our story may at least help enliven those different from ours, and vice versa. We think that part of the problem with suicide and euthanasia has been that we have all assumed we know what the notions mean, while the story that should underlie the Christian understanding of suicide and euthanasia is not that of wider society.

For example, it is often assumed that the background belief or story that displays the meaning and reasons against suicide and euthanasia is the "natural desire to live" that is grounded in our justified fear of dying or our love of life. The "natural desire to live" is thus taken to be a universal story that somehow sustains or is the basis of any particular account of suicide or euthanasia. But on reflection it is clear that there is no such universal desire, for the very meaning "to live" depends on particularistic commitments of a people's form of life. Of course, the "natural desire to live" can be interpreted as an instinct of moral significance, but when this is done we lack adequate skills to see whether and why suicide is a morally destructive practice. In an attempt to articulate the story that informs the Christian use of suicide and euthanasia we are really beginning with a very different question, namely, "Do we have an obligation to live, and if so what kind of an obligation is it?" Or perhaps more fundamentally still, "What are the moral reasons that should form our interest in continuing our existence?"

2. Memory, Community and the Reasons for Living

Most of what is important to our moral existence is not what causes us problems, but what is behind those problems and never raised as a question. Our failure to notice what we are about often makes us reach for theories to explain our moral judgments that fail to do justice to our convictions. Anthropologists and historians of religion, for example, remind us that in primitive cultures, the gravest transgressions a person can make are those that challenge or deny the sustaining story of his or her community.[11] The most disruptive practices or acts in a community are those that abandon or deny the virtues and skills which the character of a community makes available and incumbent on the members of that community. In theological terms, we call such forgetfulness "sin," as we literally forget what we are about as people who have been created by a God who sets our way.

The role of the theological ethicist is to continually call us back to and seek a greater understanding of our sustaining story and the moral skills it provides for those people called Christian. Theology, therefore, is the attempt to keep us faithful to the character (the story and skills) of our community lest we forget who and why we are. It charges the imagination by helping us to notice those images that provide convictions that will truthfully form our existence.

2.1   Memory and Community

When forgetfulness is sin, memory becomes a prized virtue. But memory cannot be understood simply along the lines of "remembering the past" or even "preserving an identity." Such "memories" can too easily become confused, are often open to widely divergent interpretations, and have the potential for being dangerously conservative. If memory is to be a useful concept in discussing ethical theory it must be distinguished from the simpler senses of "remembering."

For example, almost any American would name as crucially formative periods in our history the American Revolution and the Civil War. There is, however, a considerable difference of opinion on what these periods mean—that is, how we should remember them today. The kind of memory which truly shapes and guides a community is the kind that keeps past events in mind in a way which draws guidance from them for the future. The questions we should ask about the American Revolution and the Civil War are, "Do we want to be identified as a people with the kind of nation which fought such a revolution and such a civil war? What are the images and skills found in our stories about our past which would enable us to answer and carry out that question?"

Memory must not concentrate on events but on character, or it can become perverted into a pathological force. In a common sense way we call this situation "living in the past." The anthropologist Jules Henry has given us a dramatic illustration of this use of memory. He speaks of those people who live only through memories of past triumphs or hopes, defiantly rejecting the present or the future that does not match up to their remembrances.[12] Viewing the present through the strong images of the past, they cannot interpret their surroundings correctly. Memory has bound them to the past, warped the present, and robbed the future of reality apart from their delusions. Henry concludes by quoting Kierkegaard: "Memory is emphatically the real element of the unhappy. . . . In order that the man of hope may be able to find himself in the future, the future must have reality. . . ."[13]

The Christian should have a particular aversion to the use of memory which shuts out the future. This use of memory shows a distrust of the mercy, power and love of the God who is the source of all time and creation. For instance, Wolfhart Pannenberg speaks of man's "enmity toward the future" as sin: "When man asserts himself against the future, he misses his authentic existence, betrays his destiny to exist in full openness toward what is to be, and abdicates his participation in God's creative love."[14]

Instead of trying to understand "memory" through the model of "remembering," we should take memory to mean "being present in mind." "Presence" is the fundamental meaning of memory. We are truly present when we are living aware of the past and the future, knowing that "the present time" is only a moment's flow towards the future. When we are present, we are "fully here," and to have something "present in mind" through memory is to have it here with us in all its creative force. Memory has creative force when it reminds us not of past events but of the character which produced them, and when the memory of that character challenges us to renounce it or be true to it in the present moment.

The problem with suicide is that it eradicates the presence of the other and results in the other's loss in our memory. For we are suggesting that our very existence—that is, our willingness to be present—has moral significance that we seldom notice. It is like the importance of being physically present at a moment of grief or tragedy, and of the power and support generated toward those we love by our "mere" presence. We seldom know what to say on such occasions, but we know we should be there. In the same manner we know we must be here and be willing to die in a manner that makes it possible for us to be present in memory.

2.2   Convictions and the Cultural Configuration

Different communities will have different "stories" to keep present in memory, but none exists cut off from the wider world. If we have no convictions, our culture will provide them for us; and if our convictions are poorly understood or weakly held, the cultural configuration will override them. It is only by continual recourse to the sources of the strength of our convictions that we can articulate and hold them in the world.

This is not a concession to determinism, but the recognition of the complexity of human culture. The customs, symbols and even the values of a culture must be learned by all in order to survive in the civilization. Failure to do so is not a sign of individuality so much as of "madness," or what the culture will call madness.[15] Unless we replace our culture's convictions and reasons for action and belief with those which get their power from a different story, we will live our lives for good or evil in the sphere of the convictions and customs in which we were raised. A little reflection shows this is the case in mundane and serious areas of our lives. Witness the "fear" which most people have of snakes, the dark, or revealing intimate feelings in public. Or consider the attitudes toward sexuality from which many have felt a need to be "liberated." Or, perhaps even more fundamentally, look at our conceptions of what constitutes a normal child and the problems in having and caring for retarded children (let alone "normal" children!) which these attitudes engender.[16] The theological ethicist seeks ways to form behavior and belief by the convictions which represent faithful expressions of the story that forms our Christian character.

2.3 The Reasons for Living: Life as a Gift

Earlier we discussed the importance of attitudes toward life-taking, and said that suicide and euthanasia are properly seen not as forms of death but as the outcome of certain attitudes toward life. For the Christian the reasons for living begin with the understanding that life is a gift.

We are not our own creators. Our desire to live should be given shape in the affirmation that we are not the determiners of our life, but God is. We Christians are people who must learn to live, as we have learned that life is a gift. We thus live not as if survival is an end in itself, but rather because we know that life allows us the time and space to live in the service of God. We should view time not as something to be lived through, nor life as an end in itself, but rather see life as the gift of time enough for love.[17]

It is important that this language of "gift" not be understood as a poetic expression of a matter that could be more "literally" expressed—we mean that life *is* a gift. Recently, Eike-Henner W. Kluge has strongly objected to this language in his book, *The Practice of Death*.[18] He argues that the concept of "life as a gift" is logically incoherent because: (1) a gift that we cannot reject is not a gift, and (2) though a gift can only be given to someone, it seems here we have a case where the gift and the one receiving it are the same.

However, it is of course true that we can reject the gift of life. That was what the traditional condemnation of suicide was all about. Kluge quite rightly points out that the problem with the language of gift comes when one attempts to draw immediate ethical conclusions from it. The language of "gift of life" does not mean that life is never to be taken. Properly understood, the language of "gift of life" is not meant to direct our attention to the gift, but rather to the nature of the giver and the conditions under which it is given. Life is not a gift as an end, in and of itself. God is the giver who would have men and women have an independent existence from the source of all creation. Life is a gift exactly because the character of the giver does not require that the gift be given at all.

Secondly, Kluge fails to see that the language of gift in relation to life is an analogical term. The gift of life is not like other gifts in as much as the gift and the recipient *are* one—but that is to indicate that this is a gift that is not a property to possess (Kluge's version of the analogy), but a task to live out, a task where freedom follows upon responsibility. Indeed, the whole point of learning to talk of life as a gift is to see ourselves as not our own possession nor anyone else's. Rather we owe our existence to others who sustain us and finally to the one without whom we could not be at all. As James Gustafson suggests, the language of gift is not just a description of what God has done for us, but an indication of the way we can accept the gift of life in a non-destructive manner.

> The experience of gratitude is a pivot on which our awareness of God's goodness turns toward our life as moral men and communities. What is given is not ours to dispose of as if we created it, nor ours to use to serve only our own interests, to mutilate, wantonly destroy, and to deprive others of. Rather, if life is given in grace and freedom and love, we are to care for it and share it graciously, freely and in gratitude to him we have reason enough to seek the good of others, and are moved to do so.[19]

The Christian understanding of life as a gift of time enough for love is more fundamental for determining our stance toward life preservation than the language of sanctity or of a right-to-life. The right-to-life language has understandably been prominent among Christians today in relation to the abortion problem, but it is important to recognize that it is not the language offered by our primary convictions. If Christians use this language, they must keep in mind that they do so only as a political device since only such language offers them a way into the political discourse on this issue. We should nonetheless recognize that right-to-life talk is a foreign language for us, and that the seeming necessity of our using it is a sign of the tension we are now in with our surrounding culture.

Secondly, there is the question of whether "right-to-life" language makes conceptual sense. We probably do have a "right" not to be put to death, but it is unclear that we have a right to life. "Rights" language implies corresponding duties. It is extremely problematic whether anyone has a duty to keep me alive—to provide life-enhancing acts over and above refraining from life-taking acts.

More problematic still from a theological point of view is that rights language suggests we should be able to determine our lives, when our life will end and what we shall do with it.[20] But it is fundamental to the Christian manner that our lives are formed in terms not of what we will do with them, but of what God will do with our lives, both in our living and our dying. Life is not sacred as if we Christians had an interest in holding on to it to the last minute. Christians are a people who are formed ready to die for what they believe. Our beliefs are as precious to us as our lives—indeed, they are our lives. Life for us, therefore, is not an absolute, for that which we think gives our life form will not let us place unwarranted value on life itself.

At the very least this means that accepting the fatedness of our ending is a way of affirming the trustworthiness of God's care for us. It means I will not fight my death nor the death of others when it cannot be avoided.[21] Dying is not the tragedy, but, from our point of view, dying for the wrong thing. As H. Tristram Englehardt has suggested, what we need is "a language of finitude, a way of talking decently about the limits of human life, a way of saying why and under what circumstances death is natural."[22] Such a language would not deny that early death or painful death are matters we wish to avoid if possible, but it would give us the skill to know that our purpose is not existence but "the pursuit of a rich but finite life";[23] or in language closer to our everyday speech, it would give us the means to talk of what a "good death" involves.

In this respect we Christians must rethink our relation to modern medicine. For we have been taught that natural death means when doctors can no longer do anything for us,[24] but it may be that we must be willing to die a good deal earlier. For we may well have accepted in the medical imperative a Promethean desire to control death or extend life that is finally incompatible with our basic Christian convictions.

2.4 The Reasons for Living: The "Miracle" of Trust

Beside these theological convictions that should form our attitudes toward how we desire to live, our lives should also be formed to embody our existence as social creatures. At the same time our existence as members of the Christian community should enliven and strengthen our natural social existence. The area where this interplay can perhaps most clearly be seen can be called the "miracle" of trust.

Insofar as we are human we exist and are sustained by communities of trust and care. In his book, *The Ethical Demand,* Knud Lögstrup reminds us that "it is a characteristic of human life that we naturally trust one another.... This may indeed seem strange, but it is part of what it means to be human. Human life could scarcely exist if it were otherwise."[25] Our dependence on trust may indeed seem strange, especially to people living in modern cities, dealing with politicians and Madison Avenue. It may seem stranger still to those who have had shattering experiences of lack of trust and confidence in others close to them,[26] or have become aware of their own weakness and capability for untrustworthiness. Yet a moment's reflection will show that we do usually trust people to be honest, not to cheat us, not to crash the airplane in which we are riding, and so on.

A certain minimal level of trust is necessary for the very functioning of this social creature, the human being, but it can easily be degraded to the level of the minimal trust in gravity which makes us confident we will not fall up. It takes purpose and conviction to turn minimal trust into a positive creative force. Trust, like all aspects of human culture, is a luxurious skin stretched over the taut bones of survival.[27] We must work to create conditions for the "miracle" of positive, creative trust to occur. Of these conditions, one of the most important is our very willingness to live. It represents our continued affirmation that basic human trust has been strengthened and given positive force through the story which sustains our communities—that in spite of the danger, terrors, and apathy of this life the goodness of our communities is more basic. We exist in a network of relations that our death helps affirm symbolically. Just as we can survive because we can trust others, so should we choose to live because we also need to be counted on by others.

This can be seen in everyday life by our use of words like "sacrifice." All too often when we describe our actions for another as a sacrifice it is a sign that trust has failed, that in the absence of being able to trust another welfare "doing what we think is best for them," and having to represent our actions to ourselves and others as "a great sacrifice." Far from a sacrifice in any meaningful sense, this is at least a sign that trust has failed, and at most an effort to replace trust with a mercantile reciprocity by placing the other "in our debt." This comes to a head most dramatically at the death of another person, when we are left in a wave of guilt and responsibility as our untrustworthiness to them in life becomes clear to us in their dying. The problem of guilt at the death of one of our friends is not whether to be guilty or not, but that we be guilty for the right thing, and that our recovery from the wounds of this guilt be a sign that we have recognized the valid sacrifice so necessary to create the miracle of trust.

In this way our death itself speaks to and is constitutive of the presence and quality of trust in our community. Just as we work to live in a manner that continues our communities of trust, so we must die in a way that provides for healthful and morally sound grief for those whom we leave behind. The miracle of trust is both a reason for living and a reason for dying in one way rather than another. There is no question of denying grief at death, but rather that we die in a way that leaves behind us a morally healthy community of grief. This is what makes a proper funeral so important; it is a means of forming and expressing grief that at the same time makes the ending of grief ritually appropriate.

3. Suicide, Euthanasia and the Affirmation of Life

These theological and ethical considerations provide us the context that makes intelligible the reason that suicide has generally been prohibited, and particularly so for those who share the Christian story. The prohibition against suicide is a way of affirming how we should die in our communities in a non-destructive way for those who continue after us. It is a symbolic claim that insists we remember our primary business is about living, not dying. The moral prohibition against suicide is not meant to point a judgmental finger at the one who does or attempts to commit suicide,[28] but rather it is a notion meant to awaken us to the convictions needed to shape the character of our communities in such a way as to enhance the trust that must pertain if life is to be worth living.

Just as with suicide, we think that euthanasia should be morally prohibited. Some of the reasons for this are purely pragmatic, such as (1) knowing if a disease is really fatal; (2) the possibility of new cures being developed; (3) the difficulty of obtaining informed consent under pain or drugs; (4) legal problems with distinguishing euthanasia from murder; (5) controlling it as a medical practice and its effect on the ethos of medicine.[29]

These pragmatic reasons are important from the perspective of public policy, but they are not morally why euthanasia is rightly thought to be problematic; indeed, we suspect that euthanasia could be pragmatically controlled if we wished to do so. Rather it is a matter of not killing ourselves, even if we are in pain, as a way of affirming our continued contribution and affirmation of the goodness and care of the community in which we exist. In other words, our unwillingness to kill ourselves even under pain is an affirmation that the trust that has sustained us in health is also the trust that sustains us in illness and distress; that our existence is a gift ultimately bounded by a hope that gives us a way to go on; that the full, present memory of our Christian story is a source of strength and consolation for ourselves and our community. Community, of course, is not a warm feeling or an ever-retreating ideal. It is that group of people whose lives are shaped by a common story. Thus, "erosion of communities" is not simply the progressive blunting of our feelings of other-regardingness, though this may be involved. Rather it is the pernicious dissolution of the order, coherence and power of a story to make an issue like "other regardingness" even significant.

With this in mind, we must be especially careful that euthanasia, though often supported by the most humane arguments, does not become a way of doing away with those who bother us rather than giving them care. It may be that the demand for euthanasia comes because we lack the skills humanely to know how to be with and care for the dying, especially when we are the one doing the dying. Humans never kill more readily than when we kill in the name of mercy. We must be careful that the mercy we dispense, especially when it takes the form of ending life, is not necessary because of our original uncare.

3.1   Suicide, Euthanasia and the Erosion of Community

Suicide and euthanasia contribute to the erosion of community. They can both be signs of pathogenic abandonment, and they undermine our notions of living bravely in the face of suffering as individuals and as communities.

Pathogenic abandonment in euthanasia has been mentioned earlier; euthanasia can be a sign that our uncare has triumphed. Pathogenic abandonment in regard to suicide is more complex, and has two principal forms. From the perspective of the suicide, his or her act can be one of the most perverse forms of moral manipulation, as it abandons those left behind to their shame, guilt and grief. Suicide is something like a metaphysical "I-gotcha!" It is often an attempt to kill or wound others.

We all know that our lives are shot through with trying to gain power over others. We want power not so much for itself, but because we fear the loss of those we love and thus try to gain power to insure and protect ourselves from the loss of their love. We thus are often engaged in running exchanges of power through love and our relationships with others. Most of the time these tradeoffs are balanced out, and while they are potentially very destructive they are often simply perverse in their covertness, often even being concealed from ourselves. It is one of the messier and less noble things about being human.

Now suicide is the ultimate revenge, the unanswerable tradeoff, the metaphysical I-gotcha. There is nothing we can do to pay back the moral debt. We are left with a guilt that cannot be formed in a useful manner. Its negativity in this regard is even self-defeating, if we can speak of the defeat of a person dead by his own hand, for all that is left for those behind is to reject their guilt and in the process the memory of the one that committed suicide.

Suicide does horrible damage to memory, for it eradicates a history that is the same as the self.

Yet perhaps just as common, and certainly mingled with revenge suicide, is the pathogenic abandonment of the individual by his or her community. Many of the suicides that occur are not occasions for blaming the agent, but rather the final affirmation and sealing of a long process of abandonment by the community, the dramatic expression of an abandonment experienced across a person's lifetime. Even though we often think of suicide occurring under conditions of extreme stress or constant threat of life, Eugene Genovese reminds us in *Roll, Jordan, Roll* that slaves never committed suicide in large numbers; though abandoned by the white society, they found a sustaining faithfulness in their own community. "The assertion that slaves frequently committed suicide, quaintly put forward by some historians as a form of 'day-to-day resistance to slavery,' rests on no discernible evidence. The strong sense of stewardship in the quarters—of collective responsibility for each other—probably accounts for the low suicide rate more than does any other factor."[30]

Suicide understood against this background is a sign of failure of community. This is especially cogent in our society where "abandonment" is often called the pursuit of life, liberty and happiness, and hallowed by the ethics of individualism. We may well have a "right," within the framework of libertarian ethics, to commit suicide.

In this connection, MacIntyre reminds us that the concept of rights, which we have learned to take for granted, only emerges in the modern age:

> The central preoccupation of both ancient and medieval communities was characteristically; how may men together realize the true human good? The central preoccupation of modern men is and has been characteristically: how may we prevent men interfering with each other as each of us goes about our own concerns. The classical view begins with the community of the *polis* and with the individual viewed as having no moral identity apart from the communities of kinship and citizenship; the modern view begins with the concept of a collection of individuals and the problem of how out of and by individuals social institutions can be constructed.[31]

It is therefore not surprising, but indeed a correlative of liberal political theory that one should have the "right" to commit suicide. We must ask ourselves whether in accepting that right we have unwittingly affirmed a society that no longer wishes to provide the conditions for the miracle of trust and community.

If we are right about this, then those who would redescribe suicide as a sickness rather than a moral problem are leading us up a blind alley. To call suicide a sickness, even though some suicides may be sick, is an attempt to take the moral onus off those who commit suicide.[32] We fail to see that at the same time you take the moral onus off the society which failed to provide the forms of care and trust necessary to sustain a commitment to life.

Suicide and euthanasia also undermine our notions of what it is to live bravely in the face of suffering; they tempt us to take on a story that will pervert not only our manner of dying but of living. When this paper was given as a lecture, a man once violently objected to our position. He did so because he felt that suicide must remain a constant option, for he never wanted to grow so old that he became a burden to anyone, in particular to his children. But that is exactly our primary concern, namely, that the voluntary taking of one's own life has itself become a way of life in order to let people play out false stories of bravery and heroism, to sustain the hollow sense of sacrifice referred to earlier. There is nothing wrong with being a burden! The care of the elderly is a crucial act for witnessing our celebration of their lives and ours.

Indeed, living does require bravery. It is not, however, the bravery of ending life but of continuing it. This position obviously involves some assumptions about the moral role of suffering, i.e., suffering is not always an evil to overcome but often part of life we must learn to live with. Suffering is a highly relative matter which we should be willing to bear for the good and with the aid of the community—so we will not put our friends and lovers in the position of having to kill us. Some would fear boredom and uselessness even more than suffering. But it is not our right to end our life prematurely because we fear boredom. As Chesterton pointed out, only children, old folks and God understand how much energy it takes to sustain repetition.[33] It certainly takes extraordinary commitments to sustain our lives, but they are not different commitments from those we must make when we are young.

3.2 "Letting Die" and the Homeliness of Tragedy

Having said this we are sure that there are cases we would not describe as suicide even though they look very much like suicide, Saul and those who died at Massada having already been mentioned as examples. We are even surer that there are cases that may call for actions that look very much like euthanasia.

There is no point in keeping someone alive beyond all reason, especially when "death" is being kept at bay by means over which the agent has little control.[34] Justice demands that we give to one what we would have for all, but that may not mean we must always do everything we can do for the dying. We would question, however, if such instances are properly described as euthanasia. For here we think the distinction between putting to death and letting die makes sense. If we have entered the dying process there are times that we can actively intervene to help ourselves die. We doubt that most cases will require such active intervention. The issue at stake here is not whether we are putting ourselves to death, but rather our right to refuse medical care.[35] We do not have an obligation to use dialysis, especially when we are old and few depend on us. We have the right to die as we have lived. We would agree with any who wished to object that having said this there seems to be little difference between active intervention and refraining to give care. Yet the moral reason not to actively intervene, but rather to refrain from acting, is to show the one who suffers the continuing trustworthiness of his or her existence. Our refraining to act, or our refraining from extraordinary care, may be a symbolic act of the trustworthiness of our existence.

It seems to us that cases such as Captain Oates[36] are instructive in this respect. For what Oates did was allow those that were left alive to describe what happened as "the blizzard killed him." Their refusal to use their own hand to kill him, even in the sense of leaving him behind, was a way of symbolically gesturing their care for him.

Finally, we feel that to end one's own life, either by one's own hand or by requesting the hand of another to do it, places too great a burden on those who are left, as it asks us to cooperate in a process we should keep distant from. To ask us to passively or actively cooperate in the ending of life opens us to temptations best kept at bay—that we should determine for another whether they will live or die. To help another die invites us far too readily to justify our action by turning it into a policy, by saying that euthanasia is an act of mercy, a policy that is hard to control and even harder to adopt if we are to learn to look on life as a gift.

We are aware that our position may well result in some tragic circumstances. But then finally that is what the moral life is all about. Tragedy is a homely thing; the heart adapts and copes, if we are to live humanely.

7. The Moral Limits
of Population Control

In his novel *The Wanting Seed* Anthony Burgess describes an overpopulated society like that assumed to be our destiny by those who argue that
unless we stem the tide of population growth we will face certain disaster. For
example, the government in Burgess' overpopulated world as a means of
reducing population growth actively promotes sexual perversion. Women are
required to dress unattractively using no makeup and flattening their breasts.
Homosexuality is the rule of the day, as only homosexuals are eligible for high
government positions or for promotion in the bureaucracy. (Even being a
member of a pro-natalist family can hurt you.) Everywhere the Ministry of
Infertility, the most powerful organization in society, puts up posters showing
embracing pairs of the same sex with such legends as "It's Sapiens to be
Homo" or "Love Your Fellow-Men."

In such an overpopulated society it is of course against the law to have more
than one child and even for that one you must get a license. Moreover, this
government goes far beyond the operant conditioning techniques suggested by
our current anti-natalists such as paying people not to have children, for in
Burgess' world parents are paid if their one child meets some "accident" and
dies before he or she reaches the reproductive age. In addition, as a logical
deduction from such an ecological ethic the government pays for the death in
proportion to the amount of fertilizer that can be abstracted from the body.
Thus when the small son of the heroine of the novel, Beatrice-Joanna Foxe,
dies of a curable disease, the doctor, who made little effort to cure the child,
comforts Beatrice by suggesting that she "think of this in national terms, in
global terms. One mouth less to feed. One more half-kilo of phosphorus
pentoxide to nourish the earth. In a sense, you know, Mrs. Foxe, you'll be
getting your son back again." This proves to be but a shadow prophecy,
however, as finally cannibalism becomes the order of the day.

Many today argue that this kind of world is unavoidable unless we begin now to place stringent controls on mankind's penchant to reproduce. Yet it is interesting that Burgess uses the population issue in this novel to explore a different but related concern. For Burgess suggests that it is exactly man's assumption that he can create and control his destiny that creates the hell of a society based on the presumption that it is humane to literally eat your fellow man. Burgess' point is not the same as the semi-Luddite platitudes connected with the ecology movement about man learning his place in nature. Rather, his concern is with what he regards as the unwarranted Promethean assumptions that are embodied in our most humane endeavors. As the Prime Minister of the anti-natalist government in Burgess' novel says, they could solve the population problem tomorrow by killing off three-quarters of the world's population—"But the government is not concerned with killing but with keeping people alive. We outlawed war; we learned to predict earthquakes and conquer floods; we irrigated desert places and made the ice-caps blossom like a rose. That is progress, that is the fulfillment of the part of our liberal aspirations. . . . We removed all the old natural checks on population. The history of man is the history of the control over his environment. True, we have been let down. The greater part of mankind is not yet ready for the Pelagian ideal, but soon perhaps they may be. Perhaps very soon."

Burgess thinks, I suspect, that those who call for extreme measures for population control are but the continuation of this fundamental posture toward human existence. In other words, the very humanism that prompts the proposals to control population growth masks a perverse pretentiousness that ends by destroying humanity in its own name. A more chastened humanism correctly sees that the population issue raises a much more profound dilemma than simply the question of finding more and better ways to reduce population growth. As A. N. Hill says,

> The dilemma is this. All the impulses of decent humanity, all the dictates of religion and all the traditions of medicine insist that suffering should be relieved, curable diseases cured, preventable disease prevented. The obligation is regarded as unconditional: it is not permitted to argue that the suffering is due to folly, that the children are not wanted, that the patient's family would be happier if he died. All that may be so; but to accept it as a guide to action would lead to a degradation of standards of humanity by which civilization would be permanently and indefinitely poorer. . . . Some might (take) the purely biological view that if men will breed like rabbits they must be allowed to die like rabbits. . . . Most people would still say no. But suppose it were certain now that the pressure of increasing population, uncontrolled by disease would lead not only to widespread exhaustion of the soil and of other capital resources but also to continuing and increasing international tension and disorder, making it hard for civilization itself to survive: Would the majority of humane and reasonable people change their

minds? If ethical principles deny our right to do evil in order that good may come, are we justified in doing good when the foreseeable consequence is evil?[1]

It may be that the issues raised by Hill and Burgess can be restated in terms of the basic deontological or teleological options. However, I have begun in this way in order to suggest that ethically the issue of population control is more complex than the deontological-teleological alternative in itself reveals— or, put more accurately, these ethical options make sense only in terms of a whole set of background beliefs about the nature of human existence. For finally what is at stake in terms of the ethics of population control is what you think it worth having yourself and others die for. For Hill is right, I think, that ultimately the issue may be that if we are determined to do good we must be prepared to will our own and others' suffering and death.

With this said I want to try to do two things in this essay: (1) I want to analyze some of the issues of the public debate about population control and suggest in what ways the philosopher and ethicist may be able to shed a certain amount of light on these problems. The problem with the population issue from an ethical perspective is that in spite of the huge literature and impassioned positions surrounding it there is no immediate way of determining the kind of ethical problem that the issue should raise. This is important, for it indicates that ethics is not just a decision procedure but involves the question of how the problem is to be formulated at all—i.e., normative ethics is concerned not just with deciding what is right or wrong about already specifiable problems but with understanding why certain issues should be considered problems at all. (2) I want to try to suggest the most responsible framework for the analysis of what is at stake in the population issue.

One of the main problems running through the population debate in its popular form is the relationship of empirical claims to value opinions. Simply stated, the question of the population crisis seems to be an empirical question: namely, can it be established that there are now too many people (or that there will soon be too many) for our resources to sustain? However, even a superficial perusal of the literature surrounding this issue will reveal that there cannot be a "value free" interpretation or presentation of the so-called facts. There is no single "population problem" but rather there are many accounts of the issue that seem to have been shaped by the sensitivities, disciplines and ethical values of those who are describing the situation. Moreover, the way "the problem" is defined influences the formulation of necessary nostrums. For example, some focus on the immediate crisis of the underdeveloped nations, some on that of the developed nations, and thus stress the immediate problem of preventing more births. Others may focus on the ecological crisis and threats to our quality of life and thus recommend new patterns of consumption. Still others may dwell on the long-term issues in world-wide perspective, assessing the ultimate carrying capacity of the earth and the likelihood of the exhaustion of resources and thus try to recommend policies now for the long run. Thus not every participant in the population debate, simply because he talks of a population crisis, can be assumed to be talking about the same thing. They can differ at least in respect to (1) the subject of the population crisis (world, underdeveloped countries, developed), (2) the nature of the crisis (food, resources, ecology, war), (3) the immediacy of the crisis (now, near future, distant future) and (4) nostrums (voluntary, coercive, birth control, consumptive pattern, increased food production).

In spite of the voluminous literature surrounding these issues, I think it is fair to say that as yet there is no consensus over some fundamental questions which must be answered before any ethical judgment can be made. For example, it is a highly disputed question whether we must immediately achieve replacement level population growth if we are to eat sufficiently in the forseeable future. Of course one can always say it is not a matter of eating but of environmental deterioration that population causes, but again that is a debatable matter. For example, Barry Commoner denies that our ecological problem is intimately tied to the population issue. He points out that the increase in production has doubled the increase in population since World War II and thus he concludes that "population growth in the U.S. has only a minor influence on the intensification of environmental pollution."[2]

However, even if one grants in a loose way that we are victims of a population crisis, there is no agreement about how or who should decide what ought to be done. For, is the crisis a matter of rate or the actual size of the population;[3] how much should we be concerned with how population policies affect the age-distribution of a society?[4] Or if we need to reduce population growth, should one sector of society be singled out because of its high rate of growth, i.e., the poor, who have more children? (Early in the debate this was recommended, but it is now no longer so prominent, especially as ecological concerns have become more dominant. For the middle-class child consumes a good deal more than the many children of the poor. Ironically, the surest way of reducing a couple's reproductive habits is to make them a member of the middle class, but by doing so you only increase the ecological problem as affluence creates more waste.) Are voluntary measures (family planning) enough to stem population growth or do we need to develop "population control" programs that would not depend on voluntary compliance?[5] (Statistics do seem to bear out the contention that family planning will not stem population growth in all countries by simply eliminating unwanted children. Another irony in this debate is that of population control people identifying with the family planning movement, as the latter is really grounded in the libertarian principle of the right of each family to decide the number of children it wants.)

What must be said about these kinds of issues is that they are confusing not just to the ethicists but to the experts themselves. In other words, I am indicating that part of the reason the ethicist cannot make up his mind on these issues is that the data as yet are insufficient. Yet what is disturbing is how readily many develop extreme ethical recommendations on the basis of this kind of information. For example, many recommend abortion as a population control technique without any discussion of the ethics involved in abortion.[6] Or they recommend coercive birth control measures such as compulsory sterilization with no consideration of the violation of the rights of the individual. Or they recommend penalties against the third child such as withholding of education with no consideration of whether that is just. Some, however, feel that such measures are far too conservative and suggest that we need a whole restructuring of the family in relation to the rest of society. What must be denied is that parenthood is a right. Even "unnatural forms of sexual intercourse" should be encouraged as a means to keep down the growth of population. Finally, as the Paddocks suggest, we should as a developed nation direct our aid to the underdeveloped countries the way a battlefield hospital classifies and aids the wounded (triage), thus condemning to death those that are too far gone.[7]

The kind of assumption that lies behind these sorts of proposals has been most clearly articulated in Garrett Hardin's classic essay "The Tragedy of the Commons," where he flatly states that "Injustice is preferable to total ruin."[8] According to Hardin our situation can be compared to a pasture open to all. It is expected that each herdsman will try to keep as many cattle as possible on the commons, an arrangement that may work well for centuries because tribal wars, disease and other problems may keep the number of man and beast below the "carrying capacity" of the land. But suppose that through enlightened leadership and technological advancement you get social stability and freedom from disease. As rational beings, each herdsman tries to maximize his gain. By adding one more animal he adds another full unit to his total gain. There is a negative component, of course, as the adding of a cow creates overgrazing, but since that loss is shared by all the herdsmen the negative utility for any one herdsman's addition of an animal is only a fraction of one unit. Thus each man sensibly concludes that his good is adding another animal to the herd. "Therein is the tragedy. Each man is locked into a system that compels him to increase his herd without limit—in a world that is limited. Ruin is the destination toward which all men rush, each pursuing his own best interests in a society that believes in the freedom of the commons. Freedom in a commons brings ruin to all."

For Hardin there is no way to avoid this "tragedy" except as we deny the freedom or the right of men to determine their family size. To attempt to control population growth by appeals to conscience is in the long run irresponsible. Rather, we must opt for a coercive solution; it must be "mutual coercion, mutually agreed upon by the majority of people affected." This it seems to me is the basic kind of vision that underlies the kind of radical proposal I indicated above.

Yet there are at least two decisive objections to this kind of argument. First, it is difficult to show that we in fact face this kind of ruin in any immediate future. *The Report of the President's Commission on Population Growth and the American Future* indicates that even from a strict resource perspective it would be at least fifty years before we would face anything like the crisis suggested by Hardin and Ehrlich.[9] Of course this is not to deny that many developing countries face severe problems, even with the green revolution, that would indicate the need to develop a population policy. But it is by no means clear that there is any way that one could develop a single population policy for the world.[10] If they wish to recommend that the U.S. ought to think about its own population policy in terms of its effects on other nations this would be worthy, but it is anything but clear that this would entail the kind of coercive proposals they claim we must accept on a worldwide basis.

Basically the point that Hardin and Ehrlich are trying to make is that in certain parts of the world, the pressure of population size, rate of growth, or distribution is so severe that it may prove to be impossible to develop or maintain a level of resources necessary to sustain a good life for all persons through time. Even the severest critics of the anti-natalist position such as Ben Wattenberg suggest that "population growth must sooner or later level off. While America could support twice its current population and probably four times its current population—growth can obviously not go on forever and it is wise to understand this fact now rather than a hundred years from now. It is also wise to begin to act upon this knowledge, as indeed we have begun to act upon it."[11] This is basically the point of view adopted by the President's Commission: that if we are to sustain anything like the kind of life we now have—a life of freedom, human dignity and social welfare (and cynically our middle-class way of life)—we must begin now to develop a population policy that will not see these values destroyed under the sheer crunch of numbers.

Yet this adds quite a different dimension to the discussion, for Hardin and Ehrlich talk as if the only value at stake in the population crisis is survival. The justification for the extreme measures they suggest is the assumption that without them we will surely perish. Yet it cannot be shown that in fact we face such a crisis of survival and more importantly that even if we do face imminent death as a species that we should sacrifice all values for the one end of survival.

In the absence of such arguments the use of survival as the one dominant norm tends to open the population issue to ideological perversion—namely, that survival is asserted as the sole value through which we coerce some to insure our continued way of life and standard of living. There is no doubt that many blacks and people in developing nations understand the rhetoric of population control in this light. Richard Neuhaus, for example, has attacked the whole population-ecological argument as escapist politics for the middle class, as it gives us the warrant to ignore the hard problems of war, race, and poverty. Thus he says: "Survival as the moral purpose of American life is deceptively elitist. If in fact survival is the highest goal of individual and communal life, it invites the logic of might makes right. Hardin speaks of mutual coercion, mutually agreed upon, but the economic and political equity that can make true mutuality possible clearly does not exist. Nor are the steps toward such equity likely to be taken if a society believes it is confronted by imminent Armageddon. Who has time for programs of social justice if indeed survival is at stake?"[12] Or as Wattenberg suggests, politically the population rhetoric makes viable the rejection of child allowances, better schools, and welfare, as each encourage more children. Instead the Secretary of HEW can go forth in his best Nixonian manner and say: "Ask not what your country can do for you, ask what you can do for your country—you shall have two children, no more, no less, that is your brave social mission in America."[13]

In more theoretical terms this second objection to the kind of proposal Hardin makes involves the question of whether men want or should want to survive in all conditions. As the Hastings Center Report, *Ethics, Population and the American Tradition* suggests, the value of survival ethically has an ambiguous nature.[14] Unless human beings survive, it is impossible for them to pursue and achieve other values; existence is the indispensable condition for the realization of values. At the same time, it may be doubted that people want to exist merely to exist; they live in order to pursue goods other than that of sheer survival itself. This survival is at once the lowest and the highest value. It is the highest because it is indispensable for the realization of all other values; it is the lowest because by itself it is insufficient for anything approaching a fully human life—it must be complemented by other values such as freedom, justice and welfare.

Thus the Hastings Report argues that any population policy developed in this country must contribute to the achievement of the values, such as freedom and justice, thought to be threatened by population pressures. "The goals of a population policy should be human welfare, understood in the richest and wildest sense possible—the promotion of physical and psychological security, the achievement of legitimate human needs, desires and aspirations, and the preservation and enhancement of national goals and ideals . . . Human beings do not exist to serve population policies; population policies should exist to serve human beings."[15] It would not be worthwhile for me to attempt to summarize here how the Hastings Report tries to balance the obviously conflicting claims of these values for an ethically viable population policy. It is obvious, for example, that freedom of the individual may not be commensurate with societal welfare; how these are balanced is a matter men of good will may disagree on, but it is clearly the context in which any ethically justified population policy must be developed.

Particularly important in this respect is justice as a balancing value, since it is relatively overlooked in most discussions of the population issue, or, if it is discussed, takes the form of the utilitarian greatest good for the greatest number. If the concept of justice at least involved the idea that "inequalities are arbitrary unless it is reasonable to expect that they will work out to everyone's advantage and provided the positions and offices to which they attach, or from which they may be gained, are open to all,"[16] then plainly many of the recommendations for regulating population growth are unjust and ought not to be followed out. For example, it is plainly unjust, regardless of the crisis, to make children suffer for the good of the whole when their suffering derives from no debt they have consciously accepted or contributes little to their own good. I am thinking here in particular of the various proposals to tax or withhold services from children because they happen to be born to a family that has already exceeded the two child ideal.

It is interesting that this kind of balancing of values I am suggesting has begun to intrude into some of the later writing of the population control advocates such as Ehrlich in *How To Be A Survivor*. For example, he says that the aim of the creation of a new responsible ecological society must be to provide "a life of satisfaction for each individual." "Each individual human being must have a maximum of freedom, limited only by the boundaries where his freedoms encroach on others." Thus our "society must replace its present emphasis on materialism and consumerism. We must begin to concentrate on maximizing the growth of each individual spirit, rather than each individual bank account."[17]

It is interesting that Ehrlich commits himself so totally to the value of freedom since it is exactly that value that tends to qualify the development of the kind of population policy he thinks the times demand. Thus he plainly sees that not everyone can be left free to define wherein his own freedom lies. "People are not sufficiently aware that their freedoms are rapidly disappearing because there are more and more people."[18] Thus some freedom will have to be restrained for the sake of freedom. But Ehrlich provides no analysis that would suggest, if our freedom must be abridged, how this is to be done justly—i.e., which coercive measures fall most equitably on all portions of the population; or who and on what basis will some be allowed to pursue fulfillment in the new non-materialistic culture in preference to others. Nor does he provide any description of what freedom means when it becomes completely disembodied from what has been assumed to be fundamental forms of freedom such as the right to produce offspring. He of course can reply that freedom is not incompatible with compulsion (such as requiring everyone to be educated to a certain level), but what he must show is how the withdrawal of the right to have children will enhance our freedom. This I suspect he cannot show. (Of course the right to have children is not the same as the right to have as many as you wish.)[19]

In conclusion I want to explore the question of our obligation to future generations as the most helpful rubric ethically for discussion of this kind of issue. For, as I tried to suggest above, the primary question raised by the knowledge we now have concerning population growth implies that the nature of our future generations' existence will depend to some extent on decisions or non-decisions we begin to make now concerning population growth. The present doubling time for world population is 37 years. It may be that with the development of agriculture, better systems of population distribution, and more ingenious technologies of production, consumption and reclamation we can sustain such growth for another fifty to a hundred years. Yet it clearly cannot go on forever on a finite planet if we are to will a responsible future for our distant kin. Philosophically, however, this seems to put us in a paradoxical position, for, as certain as it seems that morally we have a responsibility to future generations, conceptually the idea is ambiguous. For to have an obligation is to attribute rights, but it seems odd to claim that those in our distant future whom we cannot expect to share a common life with should possess claims upon us. Martin Golding has argued that we normally think rights and obligations are correlative to moral community which are constituted by (1) an explicit contract between its members or (2) by the social arrangements in which each member derives benefits from the efforts of other members.[20] Yet future generations clearly cannot be included by the former condition and though future generations may derive benefits from us these benefits cannot be reciprocated, which seems to exclude the latter condition also.

Golding suggests, however, that our obligation to future generations can be correlative of what he calls our social ideal, i.e., our conception of the good life for individuals under some general characterization and which can be maintained by them as good for them in virtue of this characterization. Thus by recognizing that his (the future generation's) good is a good-to-me there is a basis for recognizing the conceptual meaningfulness of the other's claim to receive his good from me (though whether I am morally obligated is of course still an open matter). Thus "future generations are members of our moral community because, and insofar as, our social ideal is relevant to them, given what they are and their conditions of life" (p. 95). Thus it makes conceptual sense to assume that future generations, like visitors from another planet, can say: "Given your social ideal, you must acknowledge my claim, for it is relevant to me given what I am; your good is my good also" (p. 94).

In an interesting way, however, Golding argues that even though it is possible to show the conceptual basis for our obligations to future generations the conditions necessary to activate these obligations do not exist. For he thinks it is problematic that our conception of the good life (social ideal) is relevant to future generations. "It appears," he claims, "that the more remote the members of this community are, the more problematic our obligations to them become. That they are members of our moral community is highly doubtful, for we probably do not know what to desire for them" (p. 97). He continues with an even stronger claim: "That if we have an obligation to distant future generations it is an obligation not to plan for them. Not only do we not know their conditions of life, we also do not know whether they will maintain the same (or a similar) conception of the good life for man as we do. Can we even be fairly sure that the same general characterization is true both of them and us?"(pp. 97–98). Thus he concludes we would be both ethically and practically well-advised to set our sights on more immediate generations and, perhaps, solely upon our immediate posterity. "After all, even if we do have obligations to future generations, our obligations to immediate posterity are undoubtedly much clearer. The nearer the generations are to us the more likely it is that our conception of the good life is relevant to them. There is certainly enough work for us to do in discharging our responsibilities to promote a good life for them." (p. 98).

Though this argument may appear a bit bizarre, I think there is much to recommend it. For what Golding has done is assert that our obligations to those that have present existing rights cannot be set aside for claims that may exist in the future. In other language, it is a deontological check on the inability of utilitarian logic to limit the number to which the greatest good is to be applied. Thus Golding is trying to suggest that there is a peculiar madness that would have us deny the claims of basic human rights of persons now living in favor of the conditional claim which may or can be made by someone who will exist in the future. In other words, he has described the philosophical issue that underlies our vague discomfort at the suggestion that we must abort some children now in order to provide a richer life for children not yet born.

However, I think at least two rather important qualifications should be placed on Golding's argument. First there is no reason to think that the priority of claims of the living over future generations should be an absolute priority. Callahan has suggested, for example, that the claims made by the present generation should be limited to those fundamental rights—the right to security, the right to freedom necessary for us to frame and live by our own values, the right to knowledge—that we judge minimally necessary to live life with dignity. Moreover, the way we embody these rights is not morally indifferent. For example, the right to happiness might entail some entertainment but this does not mean that we have the right to ruin our lakes by filling them with oil-spilling boats. In other words, it may be that the claims of future generations bear exactly at the point where we discover that the way we exercise our rights jeopardizes the rights we now claim.[21]

The second objection I think is more decisive, for Golding's primary problem in his unexamined assumption which, in spite of his criticism of utilitarians, he continues to share with them, namely, that our obligation to future generations is primarily positive. Thus Golding says: "Obligations to future generations are essentially an obligation to produce—or attempt to produce—a desirable state of affairs for the community of the future, to promote conditions of good living for future generations."[22] But while it may be true that to try to fulfill this kind of obligation to future generations may be morally destructive of present moral claims, it is quite another matter to be obligated to try not to cause future generations harm. Our ignorance and our current moral obligations may make it impossible to work positively in their behalf; we cannot, however, claim total ignorance when it comes to knowing what might be harmful to them. At a minimum it would seem that our ignorance of the interests of future generations does not relieve us of the obligation to live in a way to make certain (1) that there will be future generations and (2) that the possibilities of those generations planning for themselves is not irrevocably destroyed by our failure to refrain from those acts which could have evil consequences for them.[23]

An objection might be made to my argument that the line between preventing harm and doing good is immensely hard to determine. I have no wish to deny this, but rather I have only a suggestion about how to control how the line is drawn. Erhlich, in developing his proposals for population control, indicates that he knows many will regard the kind of society he envisages as utopian, but he claims that "we should design for an earthly paradise. We may never achieve it, but to design for any other goal would be pointless."[24] But it is my contention that to accept such a description of the task is exactly what creates the inhumanity associated with the rhetoric of population control. It is in this context that we see the significance of Burgess' point, namely, that we should not try to create a world that frees men of the limits of our human condition, for it is exactly such a desire that creates our inhumanity. We should not try in planning for our posterity to leave them a world less dangerous, less subject to suffering, less open to death or less interesting than our own. But we should at least try, and are obligated to try, to leave them a world that is not more dangerous than our own.

8. Must a Patient Be a Person to Be a Patient? Or, My Uncle Charlie Is Not Much of a Person But He Is Still My Uncle Charlie

As a Protestant teaching at a Catholic university, I continue to learn about problems I had no idea even existed. For example, recently I was called down for referring to Catholics as "Roman Catholics." I had been working on the assumption that a Catholic was a Roman Catholic; however it was pointed out to me that this phrase appeared only with the beginning of the English reformation in order to distinguish a Roman from an Anglo-Catholic. A Catholic is not Roman, as my Irish Catholic friend emphatically reminded me, but is more properly thought of simply as a Catholic.

I recount this tale because I think it has something to do with the issue I want to raise for our consideration. For we tend to think that most of our descriptions, the way we individuate action, have a long and honored history that can be tampered with only with great hesitation. Often, however, the supposed tradition is a recent innovation that may be as misleading as it is helpful.

That is what I think may be happening with the emphasis on whether someone is or is not a "person" when this is used to determine whether or what kind of medical care a patient should receive. In the literature of past medical ethics the notion of "person" does not seem to have played a prominent role in deciding how medicine should or should not be used vis-á-vis a particular patient. Why is it then that we suddenly seem so concerned with the question of whether someone is a person? It is my hunch we have much to learn from this phenomenon as it is an indication, not that our philosophy of medicine or medical ethics is in good shape, but rather that it is in deep trouble. For it is my thesis that we are trying to put forward "person" as a

127

regulative notion to direct our health care as substitute for what only a substantive community and story can do.

However, before trying to defend this thesis, let me first illustrate how the notion of "person" is being used in relation to some of the recent issues of medical ethics. Paul Ramsey in his book, *The Patient as Person,*[1] uses the notion of person to protect the individual patient against the temptation, especially in experimental medicine, to use one patient for the good of another or society. According to Ramsey, the major issue of medical ethics is how to reconcile the welfare of the individual with the welfare of mankind when both must be served. Ramsey argues that it is necessary to emphasize the personhood of the patient in order to remind the doctor or the experimenter that his first responsibility is to his immediate patient, not mankind or even the patient's family. Thus Ramsey's emphasis on "person" is an attempt to provide the basis for what he takes to be the central ethical commitment of medicine, namely, that no man will be used as a means for the good of another. Medicine can serve mankind only as it does so through serving the individual patient.

Without the presumption of the inviolability of the "person," Ramsey thinks that we would have no basis for "informed consent" as the controlling criteria for medical therapy and experimentation. Moreover, it is only on this basis that doctors rightly see that their task is not to cure diseases, but rather to cure the person who happens to be subject to a disease. Thus, the notion of "person" functions for Ramsey as a Kantian or deontological check on what he suspects is the utilitarian bias of modern medicine.

However, the notion of "person" plays quite a different function in other literature dealing with medical ethics. In these contexts, "person" is not used primarily as a protective notion, but rather as a permissive notion that takes the moral heat off certain quandaries raised by modern medicine. It is felt if we can say with some assuredness that X, Y or Z is not a person, then our responsibility is not the same as it is to those who bear this august title.

Of course, the issue where this is most prominent is abortion. Is the fetus a human person? Supposedly on that question hangs all the law and the prophets of the morality of abortion. For if it can be shown that the fetus is not a person, as indeed I think it can be shown, then the right to the care and protection that modern medicine can provide is not due to the fetus. Indeed, the technological skill of medicine can be used to destroy such life, for its status is of no special human concern since it lacks the attribute of "personhood."

Or, for example, the issue of *when* one is a person is raised to help settle when it is morally appropriate to withdraw care from the dying. If it can be shown, for example, that a patient has moved from the status of being a person to a non-person, then it seems that many of the difficult decisions surrounding what kind and the extent of care that should be given to the dying becomes moot. For the aid that medicine can bring is directed at persons, not at the mere continuation of our bodily life. (Since I will not develop it further, however, it is worth mentioning that this view assumes a rather extreme dualism between being a person and the bodily life necessary to provide the conditions for being a person.)[2]

Or, finally, there are the issues of what kind of care should be given to defective or deformed infants in order to keep them alive. For example, Joseph Fletcher has argued that any individual who falls below the 40 I.Q. mark in a Stanford-Binet test is "Questionably a person," and if you score 20 or below you are not a person.[3] Or Michael Tooley has argued young infants, indeed, are not "persons" and, therefore, do not bear the rights necessary to make infanticide a morally questionable practice.[4] Whether, or what kind, of medical care should be given to children is determined by whether children are able to meet the demands of being a person. You may give them life-sustaining care, but in doing so you are acting strictly from the motive of charity since nothing obligates you to do so.

As I suggested at the first, I find all this rather odd, not because some of the conclusions reached by such reasoning may be against my own moral opinions, or because they entail practices that seem counter-intuitive (e.g., infanticide), but rather because I think this use of "person" tends to do violence to our language. For example, it is only seldom that we have occasion to think of ourselves as "persons"—when asked to identify myself, I do not think that I am a person, but I am Stanley Hauerwas, teacher, husband, father or, ultimately, a Texan. Nor do I often have the occasion to think of others as persons. I do sometimes say, "Now that Joe is one hell of a fine person," but so used, "person" carries no special status beyond the naming of a role. If I still lived in Texas, I would, as a matter of fact, never use such an expression, but rather say, "Now there is a good old boy."

Moreover, it is interesting to notice how abstract the language of person is in relation to our first-order moral language through which we live our lives and see the kind of issues I have mentioned above. For example, the reason that we do not use one man for another or society's good is not that we violate his "person," but rather because we have learned that it is destructive of the trust between us to do so. (Which is, in fact, Ramsey's real concern, as his case actually rests much more on his emphasis on the "covenant" between doctor and patient than on the status of the patient as a "person.") For example, it would surely make us hesitant to go to a doctor if we thought he might actually care for us only as means of caring for another. It should be noted, however, that in a different kind of society it might well be intelligible and trustworthy for the doctor rightly to expect that his patient be willing to undergo certain risks for the good of the society itself. I suspect that Ramsey's excessive concern to protect the patient from the demands of society through the agency of the doctor is due to living in an extraordinarily individualistic society where citizens share no good in common.

Even more artificial is the use of "person" to try to determine the moral decision in relation to abortion, death and the care of the defective new-born. For the issues surrounding whether an abortion should or should not be done seldom turn on the question of the status of the fetus. Rather, they involve why the mother does not want the pregnancy to continue, the conditions under which the pregnancy occurred, the social conditions into which the child would be born. The question of whether the fetus is or is not a person is almost a theoretical nicety in relation to the kind of questions that most abortion decisions actually involve.

Or, for example, when someone is dying, we seldom decide to treat or not to treat them because they have or have not yet passed some line that makes them a person or non-person. Rather, we care or do not care for them because they are Uncle Charlie, or my father, or a good friend. In the same manner, we do not care or cease to care for a child born defective because it is or is not a person. Rather, whether or how we decide to care for such a child depends on our attitude toward the having and caring for children, our perception of our role as parents, and how medicine is seen as one form of how care is to be given to children.[5] (For it may well be that we will care for such children, but this does not mean that medicine has some kind of overriding claim on being the form that such care should take.)

It might be felt that these examples assume far too easily that our common notions and stories are the primary ones for giving moral guidance in such cases. The introduction of the notion of "person" as regulatory in such matters might be an attempt to find a firmer basis than these more historically and socially contingent notions can provide. But I am suggesting that is just what the notion of "person" cannot do without seriously distorting the practices, institutions and notions that underlay how we have learned morally to display our lives. More technically, what advocates of "personhood" have failed to show is how the notion of person works in a way of life with which we wish to identify.

Yet, we feel inextricably drawn to come up with some account that will give direction to our medical practice exactly, because we sense that our more immediate moral notions never were, or are no longer, sufficient to provide such a guide. Put concretely, we are beginning to understand how much medicine depended on the moral ethos of its society to guide how it should care for children, because we are now in a period when some people no longer think simply because a child is born to them they need regard it as their child. We will not solve this kind of dilemma by trying to say what the doctor can and cannot do in such circumstances in terms of whether the child can be understood to be a "person" or not.

As Paul Ramsey suggests, we may have arrived at a time when we have achieved an unspeakable thing: a medical profession without a moral philosophy in a society without one either. Medicine, of course, still seems to carry the marks of a profession inasmuch as it seems to be a guardian of certain values—that is, the unconditional commitment to preserve life and health; the responsibility for justifying the patient's trust in the physician; and the autonomy of the physician in making judgments on others in the profession. But, as Alasdair MacIntyre has argued, these assumed virtues can quickly be turned to vices when they lack a scheme, or, in my language, a story that depends on further beliefs about the true nature of man and our true end.[6] But such a scheme is exactly what we lack, and it will not be supplied by trying to determine who is and is not a "person."

The language of "person" seems convenient to us, however, because we wish to assume that our medicine still rests on a consensus of moral beliefs. But I am suggesting that is exactly what is not the case and, in the absence of such a consensus, we will be much better off to simply admit that morally there are many different ways to practice medicine. We should, in other words, be willing to have our medicine as fragmented as our moral lives. I take this to be particularly important for Christians and Jews, as we have been under the illusion that we could morally expect medicine to embody our own standards, or, at least, standards that we could sympathize with. I suspect, however, that this may not be the case, for the story that determines how the virtues of medicine are to be displayed for us is quite different from the one claimed by the language of "person."[7] It may be then, if we are to be honest, that we should again think of the possibility of what it might mean to practice medicine befitting our convictions as Christians or Jews. Yet, there is a heavy price to be paid for the development of such a medical practice, as it may well involve training and going to doctors whose technology is less able to cure and sustain us than current medicine provides. But, then, we must decide what is more valuable, our survival or how we choose to survive.[8]

9. The Politics of Charity

1. Social Action and Charity

The most characteristic feature of recent Christian social ethics has been its renewed concern for political involvement on the part of Christians. The recovery of the social reality of the Gospel—that Christ's preaching was about a kingdom—has encouraged a new attitude, especially in the Roman Catholic context, about the Christian's involvement with the world. Christians are urged to break with the pietistic and individualistic forms of religious devotion to see that the religious life is also, if not entirely, the life of social involvement. Our cloister has become the world and its care, and our discipline our service to the poor and the weak.

This sense of the social involvement required of Christians has meant a new appreciation that the Gospel demands more than charity or philanthropy. If Christians are to serve, they must find ways to confront the underlying causes of poverty. We cannot be concerned simply with the effects of poverty and injustice, we must wage war on the systems that produce the injustice. The love that properly forces Christians into the world is not enough if our social involvement is going to be effective. For charity, when it takes the form of philanthropy, plays into the hands of the forces of injustice, as it only serves to make the injustice tolerable. Thus liberation theology aims not just to aid the poor but to give the poor the means to do something structurally about their plight.[1]

The necessity of charity not only to have a social form but to be effective has meant a new awareness in Roman Catholic social ethics of the importance of power and violence for societal change. As Reinhold Niebuhr taught, love must be joined to power if it is not to be impotent in the world. The politics of charity also requires the politics of power and the cunning to know how to use power effectively.[2]

This understanding of the politics of charity finds classic expression in the life and work of Camillo Torres. In his "A Message to Christians" (August

132

26, 1965), Torres argues that love, as Paul in Romans 13:8 suggests, is the fulfillment of the law. But Torres goes on to say that

> for this love to be genuine, it must seek to be effective. If benefice, alms, the few tuition-free schools, the few housing projects—in general, what is known as "charity"—do not succeed in feeding the hungry majority, clothing the naked, or teaching the unschooled masses, we must seek effective means to achieve the well-being of these majorities. These means will not be sought by the privileged minorities who hold power, because such effective means generally force the minorities to sacrifice their privileges. . . . Thus, power must be taken from the privileged minorities and given to the poor majorities. If this is done rapidly, it constitutes the essential characteristic of a revolution. The revolution can be a peaceful one if the minorities refrain from violent resistance. Revolution is, therefore, the way to obtain a government that will feed the hungry, clothe the naked, and teach the unschooled. Revolution will produce a government that carries out works of charity, of love for one's fellows—not only for a few but for the majority of our fellow men. This is why the revolution is not only permissible but obligatory for those Christians who see it as the only effective and far-reaching way to make the love of all people a reality. . . . After the revolution we Colombians will be aware that we are establishing a system oriented toward the love of our neighbor. The struggle is long; let us begin now.[3]

But as Torres' own life manifests, the logic of this position requires if revolution cannot come by peaceful means, the Christian in the name of charity must be willing to use a gun.

1.1 Charity and the Demand of Effectiveness

It is just such a conclusion that indicates that something has gone terribly wrong in the linking of charity with effectiveness. For while it is certainly true that the Gospel is a social gospel[4]—Jesus is the bringer of the kingdom where charity reigns—what becomes all important is *how* that kingdom is served. By linking charity with effectiveness we turn Christ's command to care for the neighbor into a general admonition of care, but what is important is *how* Christ taught us to care for the neighbor. For we must care as he cared and by the world's standard Christ was ineffective. This may mean that the most effective politics cannot be open to Christian participation exactly because the means required for effective politics are inappropriate to the kind of kingdom we serve as Christians.

Moreover, this may help us see that the politics that charity requires of us is ineffective in a significantly effective way. For example, a politics of charity rightly formed should help the world redefine what politics involves. For the politics of the world is perverted because it takes power and violence to be the essence of human and institutional relations. We Christians have no interest in denying that descriptively this is often true. Rather it is our contention that this need not be the case and thus remind the world that political life must also embody those visions of the good that men and societies should have beyond their need to survive.

For the worst thing that Christians do when they take up the means of the politics of effectiveness is they leave the world to its own devices. We, thus, serve the poor as if nothing is more important than their and our own survival. But surely that is to pervert the very heart of the Gospel from which we learn that what we have to fear is not death, but dying for the wrong thing. When charity is tied to the ethics of effectiveness, it leads us to the illusion that survival is an interesting value for Christians. We thus fail to accomplish our primary task as Christians, namely, to confront those that would secure the good through violence with the truth of the cross. In a world where the value of every action is judged by its effectiveness, it becomes an effective action to do what the world understands as useless.

1.2   Charity, Effectiveness and the Poor

This is not to deny that prominent in the Gospel and in Christian tradition has been the theme that Christians have a peculiar obligation to aid the weak. But it is one thing to say that Christians are obligated to aid the weak; it is quite another to say, as often liberation theologians do, that the great mass of the poor of the world provide an essential clue to God's action in history.[5]

For when the poor become the key to history it is assumed that the aim of the Christian is to identify with those causes that will make the weak the strong. Anyone must appreciate the passion that we must all feel for the poor—especially those of us who are inherently rich, who do not need to worry about starvation—but implied in some of these claims about the poor in those theologies that tie charity with effectiveness is the attempt to identify the natural suffering of people with the suffering that we are called to take up for Christ. In effect, this is the attempt to make the Christian life accessible without training. I am sure that the poor have a special place in God's kingdom, but I am equally sure that the Christian life involves more than being oppressed or identifying with the oppressed.

This is important as there is a tendency on the part of liberation theology to see every social-political issue as a conflict between rich and poor. For example, Richard Schaull suggests that we are currently "confronted by a new and unprecedented polarization between those who have enjoyed the benefits of the status quo and those who are most anxious to change it. Our world is divided sharply between the rich and the poor nations; and in each country a struggle is taking shape between those groups, races and classes who have awakened to their inferior position and those who are reluctant to make way for the new order. Consequently, it would seem that *social revolution* is the primary fact with which our generation will have to come to terms.'' From this analysis, Schaull concludes that the Christian must identify with the revolutionary as it is the Christian's calling to always be on the side of the poor. Thus, he says, ''If we hope to preserve the most important elements of our cultural, moral and religious heritage and to contribute to the shaping of the future, we cannot remain outside the revolutionary struggle or withdraw from it. The only path of responsibility is the one that passes through it toward whatever may lie ahead.''[6]

It is unclear whether Schaull thinks we must identify with the poor because we are obligated to do so or because they provide us with the clue to the future and thus the means for Christianity to continue to be culturally significant. Schaull thus fails to appreciate the danger of such an identification with the poor, for, as Camus observed, the slave often begins by demanding justice, but often ends by wanting to wear a crown.[7]

Moreover, to state the social ethical issue in terms of rich against the poor is to oversimplify, for it makes it appear that the only issue is to be on the side of the poor, but the crucial question is *how* we should identify and work for a more just social system. The *fact* of poverty is certainly the occasion to ask about the justice, but that is just to begin the task.

2.   Charity and the Gospel of Luke

My primary concern in this essay, therefore, is to try to suggest *how* Christians should care for the poor, that is what form our charity should take, and in what sense such a charity is politics. In this respect I am going to do a rather extraordinary thing for an ethicist; I am going to let the scripture guide my way.[8] For as I hope to show, the book of Luke contains important clues about how a politics of charity should be shaped.

In Luke we find the historical significance of Christianity, or as Luke prefers, the Way, most dramatically presented.[9] Luke knew the Gospel had gone to the Gentiles, indeed even to Rome, and it was his intent to show that this was the way God's kingdom was meant to grow. Thus the fact that dominates Luke's Gospel and Acts is that the Gentiles have been grafted onto the promise to Abraham. Christ, for Luke, is he who fulfills the prophecies of being the true Israel, and in doing so becomes the light to the nations.

Thus for Luke it is the universal Christ that fulfills not just the promise to Abraham and David, but also the promise in the creation of Adam. Thus Luke does not begin the lineage of Christ's forebears—the bearers of the promise—like Matthew with Abraham, but rather with Adam (3:28). For Luke the promise that began in Adam and was carried through Noah, Abraham, David and the prophets has again been opened to the world through Jesus of Nazareth, who turns toward Jerusalem (9:51), and whose death and resurrection sent his disciples out into the world.

2.1 A Misinterpretation of Luke's Theology of History

This view of history would seem to mean that in a fashion Christians have the key to history—that is, we know its meaning and we know where it is going. In Luke's time, when the Christians were but a small and weak minority, this claim surely appeared absurd. But from our point of view the intervening years have served to make this interpretation of Luke's theology of history plausible. For we have seen that this Jesus, this messiah of the Jews, has in fact become the universal Christ. The cross has become the symbol of an extraordinary success story.

Luke's account of history seems, therefore, to support the joining of charity and effectiveness. For the Christ we Christians serve seems to commit us to having a stake in how history comes out. And that seems to give us the warrant necessary to grasp for the means of power offered by this world. It was our destiny to take the reins of the empire from Caesar, the difference being that we will use the power to do good—that is, to be effective.

The perspective on history that Luke seems to offer has become particularly important for us because we have learned that this history that we have created—this Western Christendom—is also the history of sin, guilt and injustice. And even though we would not will injustice, we cannot become an agent in our societies and in particular an agent who wishes to do good, without benefiting from that history and injustice. The very power of Christians to do good is often built on the sinfulness of our fathers. We did not will slavery or conquest by our forefathers, yet we cannot exist without reaping the advantages of their actions. The question becomes how are we to know that, without the guilt destroying our ability to act at all.

Thus our history gives us an even more powerful reason to combine charity with power and the effectiveness it brings. For we think the way to learn to live with a wrong is to make it a right. Indeed our history has been flawed, the church has identified with the strong against the weak, but we can rectify our past by changing our history to make it come out right. In other words, our very guilt makes us require a God not just of charity but also who gives us the power to do good. We want him to be a God of love, but a love that is coupled with the power to make that love effective. The Christ who turned toward Jerusalem and whose followers ended in Rome seems to demand nothing less.

2.2 God's History and Our History

Yet I think that this is a profound misreading of Luke. For what Luke suggests is not that Christians are called to determine the meaning of history, that we have a responsibility to make history come out right, but rather that that is God's task. What God has done in Israel and Christ is the meaning of history, but that does not mean that it is the Christian's task to make subsequent events conform to God's kingdom. Rather the Christian's task is nothing other than to make the story that we find in Israel and Christ our story. We do not know how God intends to use such obedience, we simply have the confidence he will use it even if it does not appear effective to the world itself.

In this respect I think a closer look at how Luke understands God's purpose in history is extremely revealing—in other words, we need to ask what kind of story is it that we have told in Israel and Christ that should become our story. For the form of the life of Christ is the form of how God chooses to deal with the world and how he chooses for us to deal with the world.

2.3 Christ and the Weak

As we have noted, Christ for Luke is the new Adam, the universal man for whom history has its meaning. As such, it is natural to assume that Christ should have gone straight to the top—if not Caesar, at least Pilate. For after all, they are the people who can get things done, who can do something about injustice. It is they who control the legions and the economic affairs of the empire. Surely it would have made good sense to start with them. Or at least, failing there, then Jesus should have gone to the Left—the Zealots or some other group of revolutionists who opposed Caesar and Pilate.

However, instead we notice that in Luke it is emphasized that Jesus came to the poor and the sinners. Thus in answer to the Pharisee's question of why he eats and drinks with tax-gatherers Jesus says, "It is not the healthy that need a doctor, but the sick; I have not come to invite virtuous people, but to call sinners to repentance" (5:31–32). It is the story of the prodigal son that stands at the center of Luke, for Christ came and could come only to those who knew they were lost.

But even more important, Jesus in Luke is almost exclusively concerned with the poor. In Luke it is the poor who are blessed (6:20), not just those who are "poor in spirit" as Matthew has it. Moreover, it is to the poor that the good news comes (4:18, 7:22), not to those of strength or wealth. Indeed, it is exactly the latter who are in deep trouble as their wealth and strength gives them the illusion they can be safe in this world (chapter 16). Thus Christ says with no qualification, ''none of you can be a disciple of mine without parting with all his possessions'' (14:33, 12:22–34).

It would be a mistake to view these passages, as has often been done, as showing that Christ had a soft spot for sinners or the poor. Nor do these passages support any interpretation of the Christian life as primarily involving individualistic acts of charity. The game played out in the Gospel is too serious to be explained so sentimentally. Rather what we see involved in Christ's concern for the poor and the weak is *how* God chooses to deal with history, namely, through the weak. But what he does for the weak is not make them strong as the world knows strength, but rather provides us with a savior who teaches us how to be weak without regret. For that is indeed what is involved in Christ's temptations—he was offered bread, a bread that could feed the hungry; he was offered all the kingdoms of the world, the kingdoms that could bring peace—but he rejected them without regret because of the terms of the gift.

But the story that gives us the skill to be weak without regret is the same story that makes charity to the weak possible. For we cannot give charity if we think that charity is a means to renew the world—that is, if charity is justified by its effects. For we live in a world wherein charity almost always must choose between lesser evils. The crucial question is how to sustain the life of charity in a world of suffering and tragedy, that is, in a world where helping some means others cannot be helped.[10]

What we are offered in Christ is a story that helps us sustain the task of charity in a world where it can never be successful. That is why charity for Christians is not something we wish to do, it is an obligation. We are commanded to be charitable. Such a command of charity becomes possible just to the extent that we are freed from the compulsion to combine power with charity, effectiveness as the criterion and form of charitable actions. We are freed in this respect exactly because we know that charity is not required in order to justify our existence, to rid us of our guilt, but because it is the manner of being most like God. For we are commanded not to be revolutionaries, or to be world-changers, but simply to be perfect.[11]

What charity requires is not the removing of all injustice in the world, but rather meeting the need of the neighbor where we find him. Indeed it is the story of Christ that gives us the skills even to be able to see who is our neighbor. Thus

> On one occasion a lawyer came forward to put this test question to him: ''Master, what must I do to inherit eternal life?'' Jesus said, ''What is written in the Law? What is your reading of it?'' He replied, ''Love the Lord your God with all your heart, with all your soul, with all your

strength, and with all your mind; and your neighbour as yourself.'' ''That is the right answer,'' said Jesus; ''do that and you will live.''

But he wanted to vindicate himself, so he said to Jesus, ''And who is my neighbour?'' Jesus replied, ''A man was on his way from Jerusalem down to Jericho when he fell in with robbers, who stripped him, beat him, and went off leaving him half dead. It so happened that a priest was going down by the same road; but when he saw him, he went past on the other side. So too a Levite came to the place, and when he saw him went past on the other side. But a Samaritan who was making the journey came upon him, and when he saw him was moved to pity. He went up and bandaged his wounds, bathing them with oil and wine. Then he lifted him on to his own beast, brought him to an inn, and looked after him there. Next day he produced two silver pieces and gave them to the innkeeper, and said, 'Look after him; and if you spend any more, I will repay you on my way back.' Which of these three do you think was neighbour to the man who fell into the hands of the robbers?'' He answered, ''The one who showed him kindness.'' Jesus said, ''Go and do as he did.''

While they were on their way Jesus came to a village where a woman named Martha made him welcome in her home. She had a sister, Mary, who seated herself at the Lord's feet and stayed there listening to his words. Now Martha was distracted by her many tasks, so she came to him and said, ''Lord, do you not care that my sister has left me to get on with the work by myself? Tell her to come and lend a hand.'' But the Lord answered, ''Martha, Martha, you are fretting and fussing about so many things; but one thing is necessary. The part that Mary has chosen is best; and it shall not be taken away from her'' (Luke 10:25–42).

This is just our task, to go and do as the Samaritan did, for it is through such doing, a doing that may appear remarkably ineffective like Mary's inactivity, that God shows us how to serve the neighbor in a manner appropriate to his kingdom. For it is only then that we will be the kind of people that know how to pray the prayer that Jesus teaches his disciples immediately after this passage, namely,

> Father, thy name be hallowed;
> thy kingdom come.
> Give us each day our daily bread.
> And forgive us our sins,
> for we too forgive all who have done us wrong.
> And do not bring us to the test (Luke 11:2–4).

3. Charity as Politics

But does the fact that the Christian's commitment to charity begins and ends in a prayer require or at least result in a withdrawal from politics? It is my contention that rather *how* Christ forces us to be charitable requires the formation of communities that are fundamentally political. It is political in the sense that the church's primary responsibility, her first political act, is to be herself. For it is only by being such a society that the church can establish the boundaries between the world and the people called Christian necessary for the world to even understand what it means to be the world. For the primary disability of the world is it does not have the capacity to recognize itself for what it is. The church, by insisting on being nothing less than the community of charity, must force the world to face the truth of its own nature.

In this respect I think that Luke's account of the Gospel can be misleading. For one of the reasons that Luke wrote was to show that, even though Christ had been hung on the cross of political insurrection, Christianity was not subversive to the Roman Empire. Just as the Jews enjoyed religious freedom by being regarded as politically indifferent so Luke argued the Christians should also be regarded. Thus Luke has Pilate say that Jesus is guilty of no crime against the state (23:13–14) and the Roman centurion at the base of Jesus' cross declares his innocence (23:47).

And of course Luke is right that Christ was no threat to Rome as the Zealots were, for Christ refused to take up the means of violence to secure a good and even charitable end. But in another sense Rome was right to crucify Jesus and his followers, as they were far more subversive than the Zealots. Rome knew how to deal with Zealots, for the Zealots were willing to play the game by the rules set by Rome. Christianity was far more subversive, because it was constituted by a savior who defeated the powers by revealing their true powerlessness. The tyrant does not fear insurrection, as the very attempt to revolt is a compliment to his power. What the tyrant fears is those who insist that charity and humor is that which moves the world, for such virtues reveal the weakness of the tyrant's power. The character of tyrants does not change in this respect even though today we have learned to call them the "will of the majority."

3.1   The "Realization" of the
Kingdom of Charity

Thus the Christian political ethic is constituted by the tension created between church and world brought about by how Christians have been taught to take the form of Christ. This tension has often been mistakenly identified as that between an ideal, the church, and its failure to be realized, the world. In other words, the church as the harbinger of the kingdom is an ideal that the wider society is not capable of gaining. The problem with this picture of the relationship between church and world is it gives the impression that the problem with the world is that it is a potential—but not yet realized—

kingdom. The Christian's task thus becomes trying to make the unrealized the realized.

But the tension is not that between unrealized and realized ideal, for this makes us, as Christians, presume that we know what God's kingdom is like or that through our actions we might be able to bring it to actualization. The tension is not between realized and unrealized, but between truth and illusion. The church is that community that trusts the power of truth and charity and thus does not depend on any further power. The world is exactly that which knows not the truth and thus must support its illusions with the power of the sword.[12]

This is a tension that is not overcome, but rather is a characteristic of our lives. For none of us desire the truth about ourselves and we will do almost anything to avoid it. Our social orders are built on our illusions and fantasies that are all the more subtle because they have taken the appearance of truth by becoming convention.[13] Our only recourse, when such conventions are revealed as arbitrary, is to assert the absoluteness and protect them through the power offered by the state.

By construing the tension that the church establishes between herself and the world in this manner I am not trying to justify Christians' withdrawing from the world. Rather, I am attempting to remind us just how radical the Christian demand of charity is in terms of the Christian's learning how to embody it in such a world. Christians do, and are obligated to, have a concern about the societies in which they exist, but our object is not to make the world into the kingdom of truth. Rather our first object must be to form the church as the society where truth can be spoken without distortion, where charity takes the form of truth and is thus saved from the sentimental ethic of kindness for which it is so often mistaken.

Christian social ethics is often seen as what Christians can do for wider society through social action, but my claim is that we must first form ourselves as a society commensurate with the demand of charity—that is, that we be the community that is shaped by the story that sustains charity in a world where it cannot be effective. This does not mean that ineffectiveness becomes an end in itself or a mark of righteousness. We must, for example, in the interest of charity ask the state to live up to its own standards of justice—to feed the poor, clothe the naked, aid the weak—but we must never delude ourselves that the justice of the state is what is required of us as people formed by God.

3.2   Justice and Charity

In the space of this essay it is impossible to even begin to explore the issue of the relation of justice and charity. However, to avoid some misunderstandings it is at least necessary to make a few general comments about how justice and charity are interdependent. This is also necessary because by concentrating on the language of charity in this essay it may appear that Christian social ethics is entirely a matter of charity rather than justice.

However, there can be no charity without justice, for justice involves those basic obligations we owe others and ourselves that charity presupposes. In this respect justice is not simply what is possible or necessary for societal order. On such a view justice must always appear as a lesser form of charity. Nor is justice the relation with and between societal groups, and charity that which is possible only in interpersonal contexts. Justice and charity are equally personal and impersonal, as each requires ourselves and the other be regarded with respect, judgment and forgiveness. Therefore, justice is not simply an insufficient form of charity, necessary because it must deal with what is possible between self-interested groups. Nor is justice that which is minimally required, charity being reversed for all moral activity beyond our strict obligations.

Rather, justice involves those historically grounded institutions that allocate duties and protections for men to be able to coordinate their wills in relation to the goods they share or should share in common. This conception of justice obviously involves more than the recent interpretations of justice that almost totally associate justice with patterns of distribution of basic values (freedom) and material goods.[14] While I would not wish to de-emphasize the importance of distributive criteria for good societies, it is important that we remember that justice must also involve a view of the good that will necessarily form how any distributive criteria work.[15] Or put differently, it has been the mistake of recent political philosophy to make justice the fundamental criterion or virtue of social and moral life. Fellowship, friendship, loyalty and truthfulness are equally important marks for any society that strives to be good. Indeed it may be necessary even to qualify the demands of justice in order to have a society that wishes to let friendship flourish as one of its central virtues.

Therefore, charity is not those gratuitous gifts that are done even though we are not required to do them. In other words charity is not an act of supererogation that somehow goes "beyond" justice. Rather charity is, as Aquinas puts it, the form of the virtues that helps score justice as one of the virtues among others. Charity does not go beyond justice in itself, but rather helps us understand what justice requires and the forms it should take.

However, the historical forms of justice in particular societies are often less than that which Christians have learned to embody in their life together. It therefore becomes the task of the church to pioneer those institutions and practices that wider society has not learned as forms of justice. (At times it is also possible that the church can learn from society more just ways of forming life.) The church, therefore, must act as a paradigmatic community in the hope of providing some indication of what the world can be but is not.

3.3   The Church as Paradigmatic Community

For example how the economic life of the church is formed is not irrelevant to how the church acts as a social ethic in the societies in which she exists. This not only involves how Christians learn to use their possessions, but also what kinds of economic professions the community thinks it appropriate for Christians to participate in. The church must again establish that not all professions and roles of a society are open to the Christian's participation. If we did this, we might again have some sense of the moral importance of the Christian's conscientious participation in society. For the importance of participation can be appreciated only if there is significant non-participation on the part of Christians. The church must provide the space in society that gives the basis for us to be able to decide to what extent we can involve ourselves in support of our society—in effect, what kind of citizens we should be.

Moreover, the question of how the church governs herself is crucial to what kind of social ethic she is. Does the church, for example, expect and require her leaders to tell her the truth? Politics, understood as the art of the maintenance of a good society, is an art that is at the heart of being Christian. The crucial question is whether we are a determinative enough community that our politics can provide a basis for authority rather than the politics of fear. For if there is no authority that can speak from the shared loyalties of a community, then we have no recourse against those who must resort to power and force, which are often more destructive since they rule by disavowing that they are using coercion.

Finally and most crucially, how Christians care for the stranger is an essential mark of what it means to be the church. I think, for example, that it was no accident that Christians have been among the first to set up hospitals. These kinds of activities are often viewed as philanthropy and thus not dealing with the systematic forms of poverty and ill health. But such a perspective fails to see that the first object of the Christian social ethic is the kind and form of care it provides for those who have no other means to defend themselves. For part of what marks Christian convictions as true is how they teach us to see the stranger as our neighbor.

Much more could be said about how the church should function as a paradigmatic community in relation to her societal context. However, enough has been said to at least indicate why the church does not have a social ethic, but rather is a social ethic. That is, she is a social ethic inasmuch as she functions as a criteriological institution—that is, an institution that has learned to embody the form of truth that is charity as revealed in the person and work of Christ. Such a charity some may find ineffective, but it is the kind of character required of those of us who are pledged to serve the kingdom of God as he has revealed it in the Cross.

PART THREE

Children, Suffering and the Skill to Care

10. Having and Learning to Care for Retarded Children

1. Why Do We Have Retarded Children?

A recent letter to the "Wise Man's Corner" of the *St. Anthony Messenger* asked a question I suspect we have all asked, but suppressed for fear of the answer that we might give to it. It read "How does one believe in God, who is supposedly good, when there is so much unhappiness in the world? I have a mentally retarded sister who is in a state institution. On every visiting day it tears me apart to see such ugliness. I know I will never understand God's purpose in allowing these poor human beings to exist with the resulting heartbreak it causes their families every day of their lives. I do very much want to believe in God, but I guess my sister's existence has caused me to resent him. How do I believe?"[1]

There is much that is theologically naive about this letter. For example, it mistakenly assumes that God is to be held directly responsible for every unfortunate event that occurs in the world. But this kind of theological point fails to come to grips with the agony that gives birth to such letters. For we want to know why or how it is that we can learn to welcome retarded children into our lives without self-pity or false courage. The "Wise Man" attempted to answer this letter by suggesting that the writer contemplate Job and consider the many accounts of people who have had retarded children and the richness they often add to family life.

Yet while no one can deny that many families have come to see retarded children as a blessing this response fails to be sufficient. For every case that one can quote that has been morally and spiritually rewarding, another can be found that has been destructive for all the participants. In other words, I am suggesting that our attitudes about retarded children cannot be based on whether or not they enliven certain families. Rather we must ask what kind of families and communities should we be so we could welcome retarded children into our midst regardless of the happy or unhappy consequences they may bring.

Of course, some may feel to even raise the question of why and how we should learn to accept retarded children is morally and practically a bad faith question. For morally it seems to be prejudicial against those who have made tremendous sacrifices in order to raise and care for retarded children. In other words it seems to make a matter of doubt out of what they have taken to be a matter of moral necessity. Thus even to raise the question is to change the moral parameters of the case for them.

However, as I hope to show, unless we can give an answer to the question of why such children are to be welcomed into the world we will have no satisfactory moral stance that can give our care of such children moral direction. For as those who work with the retarded soon discover, caring for such children means more than simply providing them with the latest means of therapy or subjecting them to the current forms of educational or behavior-modification theory. For care is not simply "doing" things for these children, even when such "doing" involves our best technologies, but it means knowing how to be with and regard these children with the respect they demand. Thus the forms of care with which we approach these children must be guided by our basic beliefs about why we have them at all.

Practically, the question of why we have these children may seem to be nonsense because it is obvious that we cannot avoid them. But in fact this is no longer true. For techniques have been developed, e.g., amniocentesis, that will allow for the early diagnosis and abortion of many children who are suffering from various forms of retardation. Moreover, we are increasingly confronting cases today where parents are refusing life-saving surgery because the child also happens to have been born retarded. Or less dramatically, we know we have often avoided the reality of these children by unnecessary institutionalization.

It, of course, may be thought that these developments are not particularly important for Christians because our attitudes toward abortion preclude the use of amniocentesis for such purposes. Yet I want us to bracket these kinds of concerns about abortion, for I think we will learn more about ourselves, and in particular why abortion is abhorrent to Christians, if we do. For I want to try to show that even if abortion were permissible for Christians, we would still have no special or overriding reason to abort a child simply because he or she is destined to be born retarded.

This is the case because the reasons we have these children give essential clues to why we have any children. Moreover, I shall try to suggest that the presence of these retarded children provides us with important skills for how we should learn to care for and raise children not retarded. For contrary to our normal assumptions, the having of children is not a natural event, but rather one of the most highly charged moral events of our lives. The difficulty many feel at the prospect of raising a retarded child is but an indication that we have lost the substantive stories that should inform and give direction to why we have children at all. It is my purpose, therefore, to try to remind us what it is we do when we have children and why the presence of retarded children is so important for helping us understand that story.

2. Choosing Our Children

It is a common presumption that we choose or do not choose to have children. Not only do we choose to have children, but since having children has been freed from the necessity of the past, we feel we *should* make having or not having children a matter of choice. Even Catholics who refuse to use contraception still feel that they must describe having children as something they choose to do. For we are people who feel it is important that we have control of our lives, that we not be subject to fate, and one of the ways that we have such control is by choosing to have or not to have children.

Moreover, this seems to be in accordance with our basic responsibilities as parents, for biology does not make us parents. Rather parenting is a role that requires that we be concerned about the conditions into which our children are born and the kind of moral and material care that we can provide them with. Thus the church talks about the importance of "responsible parenthood" indicating that the mere production of children is not a good in itself, but that we should have children in a context that they can receive appropriate forms of care.

Yet it is unclear "how responsible" we must be before we can choose to have children. Does it mean that we must own a good house, have a secure job, and be able to send our children to college? Moreover, what moral prerequisites are required for the having of children, and are moral conditions more important than material conditions? The phrase "responsible parenthood" does little to help us negotiate these kinds of questions.

The ambiguity surrounding these questions has placed a heavy burden on parenting today. For the strong assumption that we choose our children has made us claim unwarranted responsibility for their well-being. Some even go so far as to blame themselves when their children do not get the proper genes to prevent certain aesthetic problems (baldness); or some worry about when their children should be conceived in order that their children are formed by the "best" sperm and ova. Mothers worry if they are giving their children just the right amount of love or attention. This kind of list cataloging the extraordinary commitments that some parents are willing to accept in order to justify the choice of having children can be extended almost indefinitely. For when there is no reason to have children beyond our individual choice then it seems that we must claim full responsibility or none at all. Against such a background it is clear why more and more people are deciding that they would rather not have children—it is too great a moral burden.

Even though we think we have and should exercise the physical and moral freedom to have children we have no reason, no story, which says why we should exercise this freedom to decide to have children. We thus have children because they are "fun" or because we want to continue the family name; or because our parents or society expect us to have children; or because it just seems to be something that people ought to do. But none of these, or other reasons that are often given for having children, are sufficient to provide us adequate skills for knowing what we should do with children once we have had them. We thus seem trapped to live and raise our children as if the only object is to secure for them a better basis for the acquisition of goods than we had, e.g., that they can go to a better college than we did, have a better job, home, boat, etc. In such a context, however, children end by hating the sacrifices parents have made for their welfare since they perceive the goal was not worth the sacrifice.

For the sacrifice, what we do for our children, becomes a way of claiming our children as our own. They are made our property by our choice to have them and by what we do for them—they are our product. As our product, they have no independent existence except as they are able to wrench it from us through psychological and finally physical power.

But ironically, just to the extent that we must choose our children we feel that we must also place a demand on them, namely, that they be perfect. They must be physically and psychologically perfect in order for us to justify all the energy, all the sacrifices that have gone to our choice to have and raise children. After all, who wants to go to all the trouble that children represent for an inferior product.

Morever, it is the sense that children are our total responsibility that makes some parents feel so defeated when their children do something wrong. For if the children are ours, then the natural question when they do something wrong is "Where did we go wrong?" But it is important to notice that such a question, though appearing to be a willingness to assume guilt, is an extraordinary assertion of parental power over the lives of our children. For there is no better way to control others than to claim responsibility for them.

Now I think it is exactly the notion that we choose our children, and the demand that they be perfect, that has created the difficulty of explaining why we have retarded children and moreover corrupted our child-rearing practices for normal children. I want to suggest that it is an extremely odd idea that we *choose* our children. In fact, from our having and rearing children, we know we do not so much choose them, as we discover them as gifts that are not of our making. Indeed, the notion of choosing our children is as misleading as the assumption that we decide to get married.[2]

Thus I will try to show that if the language of choice is to be used at all in describing our willingness to have children it must be qualified and controlled by the more fundamental metaphor of gift. For only when we understand that our children are gifts can we have an intelligible story that makes clear our duties to them and the form our care, and in particular the care of our children born retarded, should take.

3. The Christian Obligation to Have Children

As Christians we do not choose to have our children; nor do we have them because we cannot avoid them. This was true before and after contraception became a widespread practice. (In fact, the condemnation of contraception was an attempt to take the having of children out of the realm of necessity and make it part of the moral order.) Rather Christians (and Jews) have children because it is their duty—they are commanded to do so.

Many may find this terrible, as it seems to rob us of our freedom to decide to have or not have children. But such a criticism misses the point of why we are obligated to have children, namely, that we wish to continue and people those called into the world by a gracious God. For our having children draws on our deepest convictions that God is the Lord of this world, that in spite of all the evidence of misery in this world, it is a world and existence that we can affirm as good as long as we have the assurance that he is its creator and redeemer. That even though we know that this is an existence racked with sin and disobedience, our Lord has provided us with the skills to deal with sin, in ourselves and others, in a manner that will not destroy us or them. Children are, thus, our promissory note, our sign to present and future generations, that we Christians trust the Lord who has called us together to be his people. (This is the basis of our conviction about abortion, not that life is sacred, but that children should be regarded this way.)

The having of children is hard to make intelligible unless we are members of a people.[3] But we are not just any people: we are a people who are charged to carry the story of God who gives us the basis for our existence as his people. Thus we do not have our children because we have some obligation to keep the species intact; or because we wish to furnish our country with a population large enough to secure worldly power; but because we are pledged to exist as a Christian community.

The character of that community is therefore crucial for why and how we learn to rear our children. The Christian community is formed by the conviction that the power of this world is not the determining sway of our existence, but rather it is the power we find in the cross of Jesus Christ. Thus our willingness to have children, our obligation to have children, is one of the ways we serve this community formed by such a story, namely, children witness to our determination to exist as a people formed by the cross even though the world wishes to deny that a people can exist without the power protected and acquired through the sword.

To many such a stance will appear foolish or perhaps even immoral. For there is much that could be done that might be considered more important than having children. Children take time and energy, psychologically and physically, that prevents us from being better scholars, important businessmen, serving the poor, or attacking the structures of injustice. But it is the Christian's claim that God's kingdom is not to be built by us that gives us the patience in a world of injustice, to insist that nothing is more important than having and rearing children. We do this not because we assume our children will somehow be better than we are, but because we hope our children will choose to be the next generation of those that carry the story of God in the world. We must remember that our hope is not in our children but in the God who gives us and them grounds of hope.

Of course, this does not mean that everyone who identifies with the Christian faith is called to have children or that each of us should have as many children as we can. Rather it is to remind us that having children for Christians is a vocation—it is one of the highest callings that we can have in such a community. Some among us (and not just women) will see it as their special vocation to gain the particular skills of learning how to care for and educate children. But all of us who find ourselves members of this people called Christians recognize that this vocation is basic for however we view our own particular calling.

Moreover, this makes clear that as parents we act on the behest of our community as we raise our children. In other words, we do not raise our children to conform just to what we, the child's particular parents, think right. Rather, parents are agents of communities' commitments that both child and parents are or should be loyal to. Indeed, such commitments are the necessary condition to give the child independence from the parents, for the child as well as the parents can appeal to the community for the limits of one another's responsibilities.

That is one of the reasons that the church becomes so important if families are not to be left to their own devices. For unless the child has a community that also provides him or her with symbols of significance beyond the family, then in fact the child is at the mercy of his parents. The church, by insisting that the child is not just the parents' but that the parents have authority insofar as they are agents of the community's values, gives the necessary moral and physical space for children to gain independence from their parents.

(Indeed, one of the reasons that our children today seem so much at the mercy of their peer group is the sub-culture of youth, in its attempt to gain an institution, in the absence of the church, for protection from the good and bad will of their parents. It is the attempt to find the space not dominated by their parents, but unfortunately the teen culture is not a substantive enough institution to prevent the worst forms of manipulation.)

3.1 The Gift of Children

Once having children is put in the context of this story and the people formed by it we can see how inappropriate the language of choice is to describe our parenting. For children are not beings created by our wills—we do not choose them—but rather they are called into the world as beings separate and independent from us. They are not ours for they, like each of us, have a Father who wills them as his own prior to our choice of them.

Thus children must be seen as a gift, for they are possible exactly because we do not determine their right to exist or not to exist. Now it is important to notice that the language of gift involves an extremely interesting grammar. For gifts come to us as a given—they are not under our control. Moreover, they are not always what we want or expect and thus they necessarily have an independence from us.

Insofar as gifts are independent they do not always bring joy and surprise, but they equally may bring pain and suffering. But just such pain and suffering is the condition for their being genuine gifts, for gifts that are genuine do not just supply needs or wants, as they would then be subject to our limitations. Rather genuine gifts create needs, that is, they teach us what wants we should have, as they must remind us how limited we were without them.

Now children are basic and perhaps the most essential gifts we have because they teach us how to be. That is, they create in us the proper need to want to love and regard another. For love born of need is always manipulative love unless it is based on the regard of the other as an entity that is not in my control but who is all the more valuable because I do not control him. Children are gifts exactly because they draw our love to them while refusing to be as we wish them to be.

But just to the extent that we realize that our children are a duty can we also be freed from the excessive concern and claims of responsibility associated with our decision to have children. For contrary to contemporary assumptions duties bring freedom by helping us learn to accept the proper moral limitations of being human. We destroy ourselves and our children just to the extent that we act as if there are no such limits.

3.2 The Retarded as Gifts

Thus we must learn to accept the retarded into our lives as a peculiar and intense form of how we should regard all children. They are not, to be sure, the kind of children we would choose to have, for we would wish on no one any unnecessary suffering or pain. But they are not different from other children insofar as any child is not of our choice.

It is of course true that retarded children destroy our plans and fantasies about what we wish our children to be. They thus call us to reality quicker than most children, as they remind us that the plans we have for our children may not be commensurate with the purpose for which we have children at all. Thus these retarded children are particularly special gifts to remind us that we have children not that they be a success, not for what they may be able to do for the good and betterment of mankind, but because we are members of a people who are gathered around the table of Christ.

I want to be very clear about this. I am not suggesting that Christians should rejoice that their children are born retarded rather than normal. Rather I am suggesting that as Christians the story that informs and directs why we have children at all provides us with the skill to know how to welcome these particular children into our existence without telling ourselves self-deceiving stories about our heroism for doing so. For such heroic stories can also serve to subject the retarded child to forms of care that they should not be forced to undergo.

For example, such heroic stories can lead us to forms of sentimental care and protection that rob these children of the demands to grow as they are able. For the love of the retarded, like any love, must be hard if we are to not stifle the other in overprotective care. Or to care for these children as if they are somehow specially innocent—that is "children of God"—is to rob them of the right to be the kind of selfish, grasping and manipulative children other children have the right to be. Retarded children are not to be cared for because they are especially loving, though some of them may be, but because they are children. We forget that there is no more disparaging way to treat another than to assume that they can do nothing wrong.

But just as the retarded child is a gift like any other child, they also require special skills if we are to care for them appropriately. What is important is not that we Christians have retarded children, but that we know why and to what end we have them. To have them in order to witness to what nice people we are is only another subtle way to use them. We have them because they are children—no special reason beyond that needs to be given—but as children they present special needs that we must know how to meet responsibly. For we must know how to care for them in ways that respect their independence from us as their existence, as well as our own, is grounded in the fact that we are each called to service in God's kingdom.

4. The Care of the Retarded

How one cares for the retarded child will of course differ in terms of the kind of retardation and from child to child—no two Downs syndrome children, just like no two normal children, are the same. Moreover, I have no competency to try to suggest what kind of care or training is better than another. However, I think it is important and necessary to try to articulate some general guidelines that should govern our care of retarded children irrespective of the kind of retardation and the techniques best to deal with it.

For the great temptation in caring for the retarded, as with any child, is to make them conform to what we think they should want to be, namely, "normal." We thus often care for the retarded on the assumption that our task is to make them as much like the rest of us as we can. But as I have suggested, the very way we learn to accept these children into our lives requires us to learn to see and love them as gifts which are not at our disposal.

We must, therefore, be very careful we do not impose on them a form of life that is given birth by our frustration that they are not and cannot be like us. For example, the so-called "principle of normalization" is a valuable check against the sentimental and often cruel care of the retarded that tries to spare them the pain of learning basic skills of living. But as an ideology it tends to suggest that our aim is to make the retarded "normal." This, of course, ignores entirely that we have no clear idea of what it means to be "normal." Thus in the name of "normalcy" we stand the risk of making the retarded conform to convention because they lack the power to resist.

As Milton Mayeroff reminds us, to care for another person, in the most significant sense, is to help him grow and actualize himself.[4] That is, to care for others is to help them establish an independent existence from us—not to be under our power. "To help another person grow is at least to help him to care for something or someone apart from himself, and it involves encouraging and assisting him to find and create areas of his own in which he is able to care. Also, it is to help that other person to come to care for himself, and by becoming responsive to his own need to care to become responsible for his own life" (Mayeroff, pp. 10–11). The retarded must be cared for in a way, therefore, that they are seen to have the ability to care for others as we care for them.

To so care requires the supporting virtues of patience—for we must learn to wait even when the other fails; honesty—for we must learn how to tell the truth to the other even when it is unpleasant; trust—to let the other take the risk of the unknown; and humor—that the other knows that no mistake is a decisive defeat. Therefore, the kind of care required for learning to live with the retarded requires a substantive story that will give us the patience, honesty, trust and humor to provide them with the space to acquire such virtues of care themselves.

Such virtues and story are required for all child-rearing, but it may be that they are especially intensified in learning how to care for the retarded. For to know how to care for the retarded requires the special skill not to be overprotective. Such a skill is possible when we have the confidence that the destiny of retarded children is not finally in our hands—that they and we are both sustained by a power beyond our capacity. In the presence of such a power we have the grounds for taking the risk of caring for the retarded exactly because their existence and ours are called forth by the God we have come to know in the history of Israel and the cross of Christ. For we have learned that this power refused to sustain our existence as if our existence is an end in itself. Rather we are sustained by service to a God who asks nothing more from us than to be his people who continue to have time in the business of this world to have children, even if they are retarded.

11. The Retarded and the Criteria for the Human

1. Criteria of the Human in Recent Ethics

It is often argued that the evaluation of the development and application of new biomedical technology depends on the view one has of man. The degree one thinks man is different from other animals and in what that difference consists seems to be crucial for such issues as the prolongation of life, the limits or uses of behavior modification, and the permissibility of human experimentation. Even though the centrality of our view of man for such decisions seems obvious, how the "distinctively human" is to be understood and used is a matter of controversy. This difficulty may be an indication that there is something morally askew about the general methodological assumption that criteria for the human are required for the work of bioethics to advance. For this assumption makes us forget how inappropriate it is for the preservation of our humanity to justify the exclusion of some men from human care and concern on grounds that they fail to meet such "criteria." The appropriate moral context for raising the question of the "essentially" human should not be an attempt to determine if some men are or are not human, but rather what we must be if we are to preserve and enhance what humanity we have. In other words the question of the criteria of the human should not be raised about others but only about ourselves.

Many raise the question of the "distinctively" human in an attempt to place some limits on what they perceive as the dehumanizing potential of biomedical technology. For example, they argue that we should not try to create "better humans" through positive genetic manipulation, as these procedures violate man's dignity and capacity for self-determination. For example in *Chicago Studies* (Fall, 1972), William May argues that we should not do what we can do because:

> man does differ, and differs radically, in kind from other animals and that this difference is rooted in his capacity for conceptual thought, propo-

157

sitional speech, and self-determination. It is a difference, moreover, implicitly recognized by the majority of contemporary scientists and is affirmed in a very striking way in a comment made by Willard Gaylin, M.D., professor of psychiatry and law at Columbia University, when he wrote: "The human being is the only species capable of systematically altering its 'normal' biological system by use of its equally 'normal' intellectual capacity."

It is unclear, however, if this kind of appeal to the "distinctively" human is sufficient to place limitations on our technological powers. For example, many justify greater scientific manipulation by appealing to similar conceptions of man as the being open to constant self-modification through our capacity for self-determination.

2. Inhumane Treatment

Both sides of this debate fail to notice that their understanding of the "distinctively" human embodies values that warrant inhumane treatment toward some in our society because they do not comply with such criteria. In their enthusiasm to assert the dignity of man as either enhanced or destroyed by technology, they formulate criteria of the human that appear in our cultural context as an ideology for the strong. For example, such criteria clearly embody our assumption that man's rational and cognitive ability is what makes us human. Yet this belief is the basis for the inhumane treatment and care our society provides for the retarded, as we assume such people are fundamentally other than and foreign to the human community. Our responsibility to them extends to keeping them alive, but humanizing care beyond securing their survival is simply not warranted since they lack the essential conditions to claim the care provided for those that are "fully human." Such treatment tragically becomes a self-fulfilling prophecy as we dehumanize them through impersonal and institutional cruelty or, in some ways even more destructive, the smothering care of pity. Not to be able to think as we think, to talk as we talk, or to do as we do is to forfeit one's right to be treated with respect due to another human.

The presence of the retarded serves as a significant test case for any attempt to determine the "distinctively" human. For surely any criteria of the human that would justify less than human care for the retarded on the grounds that they fall outside the purview of our species is morally suspect. The perverse effects of such a limited sense of the human can be seen not only in the kind of care we provide for many of the retarded in our society but with the stigma we associate with retardation. To describe someone as retarded is not a technical decision based on neutral scientific data and analysis: the criteria that determine retardation have less to do with the "weakness" of the retarded than with the complexity of the demands of our society as well as our tolerance of deviation. In a society already so inhumane, we can ill afford to enshrine our inhumanity in formal criteria that putatively are presented to prevent technology's encroachment on the "essentially" human.

This argument can be made in a less dramatic way by pointing out that the criteria of the distinctively human are not simply a list of empirical characteristics. The notion of the human is a conceptualization that makes meaningful or better intelligible why we associate certain empirical features with being human at all. In other words the evidence for our particular understanding of the human is dependent on prior conceptual and normative commitments that must be justified philosophically and ethically, since it cannot be assumed that the "empirical" conditions we have learned to associate with being man are necessary to the human conceptually and normatively understood. As James Gustafson has said, "A pre-judgment about what is and is not 'truly human' probably lurks in the judgment about what data to use in describing the human." Therefore, to raise the question of the criteria of the human is not first an empirical question, but a conceptual-moral claim about how the nature of man should be understood. We wrongly assume that what our eyes perceive as "normal" is what we should morally understand men to be qua human. The presence of the retarded helps us feel the oddness and the problematic nature of this assumption and its attendant ethical implications.

3. Fletcher's Position

The significance of this argument can be illustrated by contrasting it with Joseph Fletcher's attempt to provide the biomedical decision maker with a profile of the human in operational terms (*The Hastings Center Report,* November 1972). Fletcher's "profile" includes fifteen positive and five negative propositions that are meant to provide necessary and sufficient grounds for attributing the status of human to another. To be man we must be capable of self-awareness, self-control, have a sense of time, futurity and past, be capable of relating to others, show concern for others, be able to communicate, exert control over our existence, be curious, be open to changes, have a proper balance of rationality and feeling, and have a unique identity. Negatively, men are not any of the following: anti-artificial, essentially parents, sexual, worshipers, or a bundle of rights. I am sure each of will have our special problem with one or more of these criteria especially as some seem to make recommendations about how to be a good or mature man rather than the minimal conditions necessary to be a man. However, it is not my purpose to try to evaluate each of these "criteria" separately, as I am interested in trying to make a more general point concerning the vagueness of this list. For Fletcher claims to have developed a list of "operational" criteria that are empirically specifiable, but all the conditions listed have only the vaguest empirical correlates. For example, what "empirical" signs could be given as a necessary warrant to demonstrate that someone had control over himself that would be useful to the doctor?

The issue is complicated by Fletcher's failure to distinguish between criteria that are necessary and those that are sufficient to determine the human. For example, if a criterion such as having a proper balance between rationality and feeling is a necessary condition for being human, then I suspect some of us are in perpetual peril of losing our status as humans. However, Fletcher does identify minimal intelligence provided by the neo-cortical function as *the* necessary empirical condition on which all these other characteristics depend. "In a way," he says, "this is the cardinal indicator, the one all the others are hinged upon. Before cerebration is in play, or with its end, in the absence of the synthesizing function of the cerebral cortex, the *person* is nonexistent. Such individuals are objects but not subjects" (p. 3). Fletcher's emphasis on this aspect of our physiology rests on his assumption that to be human is to be rational, or in his language, "*Homo* is indeed *sapiens,* in order to be *homo.* The *ratio,* in another turn of speech, is what makes a person of the *vita.* Mere biological life, before minimal intelligence is achieved or after it is lost irretrievably, is without personal status" (p. 1). Thus for Fletcher any individual who falls below the I.Q. 40-mark in a Stanford-Binet test is "questionably a person," and if you score 20 or below you are not a person.

Before raising the more substantive issues about Fletcher's position, there are some empirical issues that should be considered. It is interesting that Fletcher places such great faith in the Stanford-Binet test, since it is extremely unclear what such a test measures (even psychologists are not all sure what intelligence involves or how the Stanford-Binet relates to intelligence). Therefore, even on empirical grounds it is not clear that the one operational criterion Fletcher gives to mark off the human is anything less than arbitrary. More troublesome than this is what empirical features Fletcher would associate with the absence of neo-cortical function, since it could involve anything from the loss of an EEG to the beginnings of senility. Fletcher seems to base his position in this respect on the assumption that activities such as instrumental learning and cognition reside entirely in the neo-cortex, but this has not yet been decisively established. Of course, no one would wish to deny the significance of the neo-cortex for our behavior, yet we should at least be aware that the identification of brain and mind is fraught with philosophical and empirical difficulties. Recent research suggests that we must be careful how we draw the distinction between body and mind, since it may be that our spirit and individuality is more dependent on "mere biological or bodily processes" than we had thought.

4. Purpose of Criteria

More substantively it can be asked what purpose Fletcher's criteria are to serve—that is, what conclusions should be drawn from them and what tasks should we try to perform with them? They seem to lend themselves to an interpretation that would exclude many that are now receiving care as human beings. Should we cease trying to obtain better living and learning conditions for the profoundly and moderately retarded? What should be done with the elderly who are no longer able to meet the criteria of being members of the Pepsi-generation? Should we cease developing resources for the care of those whose intelligence is not up to coping with our modern society because they place a drain on our resources while not contributing to the services or artifacts of our civilization?

This "profile" of man does not, I suspect, provide operational criteria any doctor would recognize, but it is rather a statement of the working assumptions about the value of human life that are alive in our culture. The strong stress on the value of intelligence as the necessary condition for all human activity faithfully mirrors the loyalties of our society. Intelligence, however, is not an end in itself, nor is our ability to reason sufficient to make us human if being human has anything to do with being humane. To assert such criteria as necessary to be human separated from the values and community for which they exist is to risk perversions we can scarcely afford in a world that already condemns some children to miserable existence because they cannot exercise "problem-solving" intelligence. We fail to notice that such criteria are really goals through which we manipulate and destroy some for the good of the "normal." The important moral question is not whether the retarded meet or should meet "criteria of the human" we have established, but whether we do not become inhuman by being concerned with such judgments rather than providing the retarded with respect and care.

Our society's high value of rationality tends to make us forget that our ability to think cannot be separated from our nature as social beings. As G. H. Mead taught, we would never be able to distinguish the "me" and the "not me," the bedrock of awareness and reason, if we were not graced with the presence of the other. This descriptive point provides the basis for the more substantive ethical claim that our capacity to reason rightly is a correlative of our ability to regard others with respect. The use of the criterion of intelligence to warrant the exclusion of those that repel and think differently from us is to cut off the moral basis of our ability to be rational at all. Put in more traditional terminology, our rational ability is not the prior principle of our moral activity, for we are able to reason because we are fundamentally social beings. To emphasize our rational ability separated from its social-moral context is to intellectualize arbitrarily the power of cognition and language.

5. Being Human

To be a man is to be able to perceive and respond to other men with recognition of care. It is unclear to me what empirical criteria are correlative of this understanding of man since the forms of response are rich and varied. That we need to develop some empirical rules of thumb to check our arbitrariness in some of the hard cases occasioned by our increased technological skill is not in question. As Eric Cassell suggests, "The function of morality in medicine is no longer simply to protect the weak and the sick from indifference or venality, but to protect them also from mercy grown overwhelming by technological advance." However, the development of such rules of thumb must be developed with the kind of exactness that such cases entail, rather than with the generality that opens them to the perversion of justifying our uncare of those who do not fit our current standards of "fully human."

In this respect, I think a strong cautionary note needs to be interjected about developing criteria of the human that will somehow relieve us of the hard choices that we are confronting in modern medicine. For criteria that are sufficient for all the kinds of cases we confront will be so vague that their concrete implications will be ambiguous at best. Even if you try to make such criteria more operational for the doctor by tying them to empirical characteristics, it is by no means clear that the moral questions involved in many of these cases will be any more resolvable. For even though such criteria may help you decide that this life is not "fully human," the question of whether care should be given still remains. I suspect that we are human exactly to the extent we can reach out and provide care for those who have no "right" to it. Put more concretely, as important as criteria are to inform decisions, we cannot make them do all the work of ethical judgment and argument for all cases, since no criterion is going to relieve or should make less troublesome the burden of deciding to operate to save the life of a severely retarded child. To try to substitute "impersonal criteria" for what should be the moral agony of such decisions is already to sacrifice more of our humanity than we can stand.

Finally, I think we should feel more the oddness of trying to determine this or that as *the* criterion that makes us human. The conditions of being human form a far too complex pattern to ever be reduced to something like "criteria." Too quick appeals to the mystery of being human can be but excuses for cloudy and sloppy thinking that attempts to evade some of the hard issues we are confronting, but they may also be profound responses to the human sense that ultimately we are not our own creators. To be a man is to be open to the call of what we are not, and there is therefore no chance that our humanity will be enhanced by excluding from our ranks those who do not understand as we. We must therefore approach the attempt to develop criteria of the human with the humility that recognizes that we would be less than human if we did not recognize that there are limits to what can be brought under our control.

12. Suffering, Medical Ethics and the Retarded Child

Certain areas of contemporary medicine are important for medical ethics because they raise in a particularly intense and fruitful form issues that cut across the general practice of medicine. For instance, the development of amniocentesis and various procedures for keeping alive children previously considered hopelessly ill have made fetal care and neonatology very interesting for ethical reflection. The cases confronted in these areas reveal the simplistic character of many moral guidelines which have been generally accepted in medical practice. The doctor, for example, has traditionally assumed he should always act to relieve suffering. But it is becoming increasingly apparent that such a principle is simply not sufficient for dealing with issues like whether retarded children should be born or cared for. Or put more strongly, we are learning that the principle enjoining the doctor always to relieve suffering, when unqualifiedly accepted, has implications which are anything but life-enhancing.

Let me illustrate these remarks by discussing some cases that are prevalent today in fetal and neonatal medicine. When a woman undergoes amniocentesis and discovers that the fetus has Downs Syndrome, a common conclusion is that the fetus should be aborted. The decision to abort is often justified as necessary to spare such children and their families a life of suffering, embarrassment and discrimination. (I realize that other kinds of reasons can be given for not having such children that raise other kinds of moral issues. However, I cannot help but feel our assumptions about suffering underlie much of our gut responses about having and allowing such children to be born.) Thus the doctor's assumption that he should always act to relieve suffering seems to support such a decision. But upon reflection this is an odd application, for traditionally the principle to relieve suffering has been understood as enhancing life. The transformation of the principle in this context to one of life-denial demonstrates how quickly abstract principles can be reinterpreted when they become divorced from their customary uses.

164

This kind of problem indicates the complexity involved in reflection on medical ethics. The renewed interest in medical ethics is encouraging, but we cannot assume this will result in the development of clear and unambiguous guidelines for medical practice. For principles are only summary statements of the values and inherited moral wisdom shared by the community or profession about the nature of human existence. Useful though principles are, they easily can be and are divorced from the original insights that gave them substance, forming ideologies for quite a different set of practices. This is why the moral commitments doctors often embody in practice are frequently more substantive than the principles they explicitly invoke. The problem is, however, that no practice can be sustained which is not properly mirrored in language and ritual. Probably one reason why medical ethics is becoming important is the necessity doctors are feeling to learn the moral language of their art. Inability to articulate the language is finally failure to practice medicine morally.

Doctors' adherence to the principle of alleviating suffering provides a good illustration of why they must understand how the principle works in relation to other basic commitments in medical practice, as well as knowing what the principle itself means. Although doctors in the past have claimed to act as if the obligation to relieve suffering were unqualified, in actual practice the principle functioned as a limited obligation. It has always been regarded legitimate to ask patients to endure limited forms of pain and suffering in order to regain health. Thus the principle requiring the doctor to alleviate suffering has been, in fact, morally qualified by the physician's conception of health and the therapy necessary to achieve it.

The medical profession has generally assumed that "health" should be understood primarily as the normal functioning of the physical and physiological aspects of our being. "Psychological" considerations have been taken into account insofar as they have a bearing on the patient's physical condition. By assuming that a retarded child ought to be aborted to spare it and the family suffering, however, the doctor is accepting an immensely broadened meaning of "suffering" and "pain." (Not to mention that in such circumstances the difficult problem of *who is the patient* is raised!) What the retarded child and its family are now to be spared are the difficulties occasioned by an indifferent and cruel society which rejects those who fail to meet its requirements for "normality." That is a far cry from the traditional concept of the suffering which the physician is pledged to alleviate.

It is questionable whether medicine can accept this enlarged sense of relieving "suffering" without being perverted. For in contemporary society it is not only retarded persons who face the suffering which comes from embarrassing, annoying, frightening or threatening those who regard themselves and their way of life as "normal." If the medical profession is willing to serve a certain societal ethos in relation to those diagnosed as retarded, why should it not use its technical power against other groups which deviate from the society's accepted standards? A doctor's commitment to alleviate suffering can readily be deflected and co-opted for highly questionable purposes in a society which identifies suffering with psychological and economic discomfort. It is all too easy to fail to notice that in the name of sparing others suffering one must justify a Promethean presumption to control and determine their very existence. The greatest evils are, of course, always perpetrated on others in the name of "their own good." Viewed in this perspective, a doctor's traditional commitment to the physical appears as a substantial moral value which protects his art from the arbitrariness of societal norms.

The care of the retarded child, however, is perhaps not the hardest one for exploring the limits of the principle of the alleviation of suffering and the practice associated with it. Cases of children born with grave abnormalities raise the issue in a different and perhaps more intense form. For it is possible to have a prognosis for these children which gives accurate information regarding the physical suffering they will undergo for what may be at best only a few years of life. It seems a natural and human question to ask why we should not be willing to let such children die in order to spare them this futile agony?

A first response to such a question might be to deny that there is any one principle which can provide an answer to it. Principles, even understood as rules of thumb, tend to assume an independent existence. When they are too consistently applied, they generally result in inhumanity. For the principle gives us an illusion of objectivity and impartiality in an area where we best not forget we are fallible and often arbitrary beings. Letting one severely deformed infant die to relieve suffering should not establish a rule for all subsequent cases; such a rule would only close off life-giving opportunities for the future. I suspect many doctors working in neonatal wards tend to preserve the distinction between "letting die" and "putting to death" because they fear the latter description would require giving general reasons for their action which might limit their choice for future cases. The distinction between "letting die" and "putting to death" relies heavily on the assumption that in such cases there is a real difference between refraining to give care and acting to end a life. The doctor knows well, however, that by "refraining" to give care he is putting the child to death. He refuses to describe it as such because as a doctor he fears the implications such a description might have for the care of future patients. This may suggest that even though in certain circumstances acting to put to death is not descriptively easily distinguished from refraining to act there are good moral reasons to maintain the distinction in order to enforce the doctor's commitment to save life. If this is the case, however, it is extremely important that we develop criteria for the careful use of the distinction.

It is unhappily true that for many children the most humane response is to protect them from a mercy grown overwhelming by technological advances that can sustain their life beyond any good end. However, in such cases we must be careful to be clear whose suffering we are most concerned to end— the patient's physical and mental pain or our pain occasioned by having to be next to a patient we cannot relieve. We should never overlook the threat we feel at having to be near those who suffer, even if it is the suffering or assumed future suffering of a new-born. In such circumstances our very humanity can be transformed into inhumanity as we recoil in hate against the other for revealing our helplessness. Our very humanity can force us to dehumanize the sufferer, because he reminds us too strongly of the fragility of the human condition. Such dehumanization is but the first step toward elimination.

Ironically, in order to spare the other person suffering we may be willing literally to deny him existence. But why should we assume that existence is only valuable when it is free of suffering? Why should we assume that we should always try to spare the other suffering when we know that often the good we do comes only because we were willing to endure pain? It is hard to calculate the importance of these questions for medical practice. If we assume that we ought always to deal with suffering by elimination, then there is nothing that can force the imagination to develop new forms of care and cure.

Medicine advances because doctors and others in helping professions have been willing to allow others to endure pain. By our willingness to stand in the presence of such pain we create the conditions that impel the imagination to explore yet unthought forms of care. Not to be willing to witness suffering makes it too easy to forget that the patient and not the disease is the object of the doctor's care. Such a tendency can be illustrated in the way we refer to retarded people as "retardates" or "mongoloids," thereby seeing abstractions rather than individuals afflicted with Downs Syndrome. When we class them as "mongoloids," we forget that a person is more than a disease; and this may lead to the assumption that in trying to eliminate such diseases it is incidental if we must also eliminate the person. Progress toward better care for persons so afflicted will be made, however, if we do not forget that these are people—suffering people to be sure—who claim our attention and care even if we cannot "cure" their affliction or protect them against suffering. The task of the doctor is not simply to alleviate suffering. He must stand before those who suffer without denying their being.

The doctor's task is to provide care even when such care may involve the patient in suffering. Of course, there are limits to the ability of doctors to act in this fashion. Cases where parents refuse to allow life-saving surgery on their retarded or deformed children are the most dramatic instances of this kind of problem. It may be that in the absence of societal support for such children we cannot argue that the parents or the doctors have an obligation to perform surgery in such circumstances. However, what is not clear about such cases is why the parents have been relieved from the burden of care for the child until it dies. Doctors have no responsibility to watch the child die in the name of sparing the parents suffering; nor should they accept such responsibility, for otherwise the parents have no sense of the full reality of the decision they have made. The doctor's willingness to protect the parents from the death of these children unwittingly supports a societal ethos that would eliminate rather than care for those that cause us discomfort. It may seem excessively cruel to ask parents who decide not to give a retarded child care to take it home, but otherwise the medical profession too easily protects our society from the knowledge that we do not care to protect the life of these children.

It is perhaps necessary in conclusion to forestall misunderstanding. I am not suggesting that suffering should be sought for its own sake; or that suffering should be accepted as a way of becoming good. I have no sympathy for some religious and philosophical traditions that make suffering an inherent good. Rather I am trying to suggest that though suffering is not to be sought, neither must we assume it should always be avoided. Often we achieve the good only because we are willing to endure in ourselves and others an existence of suffering and pain.

13. The Demands and Limits of Care: On the Moral Dilemma of Neonatal Intensive Care

1. Dilemma, Decision and Description

Time magazine describes the dilemma this way: "Should lives of retarded infants or those with multiple birth defects be prolonged—at great cost in manpower, money and anguish—especially if the life that is preserved will almost certainly be one of pain or merely vegetable-like existence?"[1] The dilemma so stated encourages us to frame a response that answers the dilemma on one side or the other: namely, should we keep such children alive or should we withdraw care? Ethical reflection, if it is to help men struggle with such an issue, would necessarily seem to be a decision procedure to help us choose between these alternatives.

Moreover, there are models of ethical reflection that seem to provide the means to respond to such a practical inquiry. For example, a consequentialist would suggest that we ought to act in a manner that the greatest good be done. The right response to such a dilemma would be the one which produces the best consequences for all concerned. An ethical formalist, on the other hand, would argue that we ought to act in a manner that our action will be consistent with the fundamental principles of moral behavior. For the formalist such decisions should not be determined by a consequential analysis, but rather in terms of general rules or principles.

It is my contention, however, that it is misleading to assume that ethical reflection should focus on decision making. The consequentialist and formalist both mislead as they seem to be responding to the question, "What should we do?" when in fact they are actually offering a redescription of the situation. For prior to the question of "What should we do?" is the question of "How do we know that we are describing the situation correctly?" By starting with the practical question—"What should we do?"—we tend to forget that moral situations do not come into our lives as given. Unlike mud puddles, situations are not something that we simply fall into. Situations and the decisions we make about them are what they are because of the presumptions we hold and how we have come to see them.

The kind of agent we are and the kinds of institutions and practices in which we are involved determine the kinds of cases we confront. Situations are correlative of the ways we have learned to see, and seeing depends on the language we use and the expectations we have encouraged through our character and roles.[2] A man's role determines the sort of descriptions we think appropriate about situations he confronts. If a policeman and I walked into a bank that was being robbed, it might be proper to say that the policeman failed to stop the robbery, whereas a similar description would hardly be appropriate to describe my activity in the situation.

Ethical reflection, therefore, cannot concern itself exclusively with what we ought to do in certain dilemmas. It must be equally concerned about how we ought to see and understand what the dilemma is. We do not come to see just by looking; we must be trained to see rightly. Moreover, one of the more persistent demands of our moral existence is to see the world in a manner that reinforces our self-concepts and roles. To be a man is to be a lover of illusion. Self-deception seems to be our fate in the measure that our lives always involve more than our roles will allow.[3] We succeed in deceiving ourselves not so much because we are evil, but rather because we fear that the truth will destroy what good we do.

These very general remarks will prove useful for reflecting on the kind of problems we are currently facing in neonatal medicine, for I suspect we are being tempted, for some good reasons, to misdescribe what we must do or not do for some children. Hence the major thrust of this paper is directed at understanding the kind of dilemma in which such births involve us. I am convinced that we will only be able to make headway on the question of "What ought we to do?" if we first concern ourselves with an analysis of how we should understand the kinds of commitments that are involved in the medical care of children.[4]

2. Care for Children: A Preliminary Discussion

The choices we confront in neonatal medicine often seem to be extremely cruel. Sometimes keeping a child alive can only further damage his or her brain. Whatever we do in such cases seems best described as a lesser evil rather than doing good. Yet I think this is somewhat misleading, for we forget that such choices are being forced upon us exactly because of our commitment to care and protect children. In fact, our charity has been amplified by an overwhelming technology that threatens the very presumptions of that care.

We can easily overlook how recently parents have considered themselves to be responsible for maintaining the lives of their children. Infanticide for children malformed or of the wrong sex has been the rule in much of human history and culture. To be sure, in recent times we have often done this indirectly by sending these children to homes that meant certain death, but our purpose was no less direct. The Nuer tribe in Africa, for example, simply assumes that infants born with deformities or other anomalies are really hip-popotamuses born to humans by accident. In this case the prescribed action is clear: put them in the river where they belong.[5] Societies have usually found a way to regard certain children as "hippopotamuses" and thus justified similar appropriate action.

For a variety of reasons, however, parents today presume it is their duty to care for their child, regardless of the child's genetic condition. John Fletcher attributes this attitude to a better understanding of the genetic, environmental and other factors causing these defects.[6] Some moral assessments regarding the status of each individual are also at work in bolstering these postures of care for defective newborns.

Doctors and medicine have become the extension of this parental commitment by providing the means to care for children that at one time, indeed a relatively short time ago, would have entered life with no alternative other than death. The development of intensive care neonatal units represents the technological expansion of this care. Of course, this development has also been occasioned by the doctors' urge to expand the research capabilities of their science. (Some babies may well be kept alive because they provide an opportunity for the resident to gain experience and perfect his craft for future patients.) However, this aspect of medicine should not make us forget that the expansion of new-born care is based on the moral commitment of parents to care for their children.

It is interesting to note how technology expands our care, for on the whole doctors do not develop their technological capacity by design. Doctors rather seek new means of care in order to meet the needs of this patient or this kind of problem. However, experience shows that this process often culminates in a technology whose range quite surpasses the original intentions. This very fact raises the question whether the new technology should be applied to this unexpectedly enlarged class of patients. I suspect, however, that there is no way to avoid the issue if our medicine is to remain patient-centered.

It is this peculiarly expansionist quality of technological extension of care which raises the excruciating problems that we currently face in neonatal units. We now face the question whether we should keep some of these children alive, as the quality of their life and severity of their disabilities turn their continued existence into a life of suffering. Our technologically expanded care has placed choices before us that seem inconsistent with our original intentions of care.

2.1   The Problem of Care

Once the "dilemma" is described against this background of care, it is easier to see that the question "What should we do?" is not one question but many. We must now ask why we assume that any kind of medical care should be given to these children at all. Why, for example, has it become a normal procedure to respirate nearly all infants that require it at birth? This is often done because it is necessary to get the infant "going" in order to buy time to make a reasonable diagnosis. Yet keeping the child going increases our expectations of saving the child. The more we give care to see if we should give care at all, the more we find ourselves committed to giving more and more care.

This suggests that doctors should take special care how they describe to the parents what they are doing: namely, that they are not saving the child, but they are sustaining life as best they can in order to have some sense of what is wrong with the child. Beginning care on the assumption that the doctor is curing the patient raises expectations in doctors, nurses and parents that makes it hard to terminate care because terminating can be taken to mean that we are ceasing to care. Later I shall want to question our assumption that the only way to care is to cure. The model of what it means to be a doctor may have been programmed too closely to producing results—i.e., healthy persons—rather than to scouting opportunities for care when curing is not possible.

Of course there are questions beyond these. Are the defects some children have so debilitating that they are disqualified from therapy? Does the fact that a child shows signs of retardation mean that it should be denied medical care? To what extent should the ability of the family to support the child emotionally and financially determine the amount of care that is given?

We cannot avoid asking who should decide whether or not care is to be given. Paul Ramsey correctly reminds us that the "What" question should be decided prior to "Who," but the "Who" often provided valuable clues to "What" should be decided.[7] We assume that parents should be primary decision makers in such a context. Yet they are often dealing with extremely complex sets of emotions involving rejection, guilt and self-blame all at once.[8] What kind of counseling should parents receive who have to make such decisions? No counseling can be value-neutral at a time like this. Should parents, for example, be encouraged to accept their child because they do not have the right to determine the life or death of their children? Or should they be told it is up to them, since the choice is morally indifferent?

What ought we expect of the doctor in such situations?[9] Should he normally acquiesce to the wishes of the parents? Most doctors feel responsible to present to the parents the relevant information and to describe the alternatives as clearly as possible. This assumes that the doctor can assume a neutral role as he simply tries to give the parents the information in a manner that they can make an informed decision. Yet doctors know that there is in fact no neutral way to describe the situation with its alternatives to the parents. The doctor's own attitudes toward the retarded cannot be separated from the way he informs the parents. And the doctor's manner of describing the situation, together with alternatives he suggests, determine to a large extent what will or will not be done.[10]

We must go on to ask what role society should play in such cases. The state obviously has an interest in how parents deal with their children. Child-battering is against the law. But should the state also have an interest in the kind of aid that parents are required to give to their children, even defective children, in order to keep them alive?[11] There are, of course, negative measures which the state might take concerning children. But does the state also have positive duties to such children, their parents, and their doctors? Should the state offer institutional forms of care for such children for their training and basic needs? If the state limits the parents' unwillingness to care for such children, what kind of aid should it give doctors to act independently of parents' wishes?

2.2 Two Possible Responses

These are obviously hard questions for which there are no immediate "right answers." We fear even raising them for they seem to invite answers that implicate us far beyond the contexts envisaged by the original question. To ask these questions explicitly gives them too much exposure. We prefer to stumble on, hoping that things will work out better than if we try to subject these issues to reflection or community pressures. Like a couple who have long since quit loving one another, yet fear admitting it lest that very admission would imply decisions that both fear, we continue on in the hope that something magic will set things aright.

Whether we raise them or not, however, these questions are being answered in practice. Moreover, some answers are beginning to be formulated that attempt to meet the fundamental dilemma with which we started. One suggests that such children should not be considered human—i.e., that these new-borns, like the fetus, do not possess the characteristics required to be treated as human beings. Thus the care that these children receive should not be of the same type as that received by those who are fully normal.[12] Another response distinguishes putting such children to death from merely letting them die. By refraining from giving them care, we are not called upon to justify our action as if we were putting them to death. In the words of Duff and Campbell we are simply finding a way to seek "early death as a management option" for these children.[13] I want to consider how both these suggestions tend to redescribe the dilemma in a way calculated to remove the moral agony from these decisions. To do so, of course, is to mislead in a specific way, and to offer effective support for self-deception.

3.   Are Defective Newborns Human Persons?[14]

Before we can address ourselves to this question we must answer a prior question: Are any newborns human persons? All newborns, whether defective or not, have little capacity for self-determination, for self-reflection, and no perceptible ability to talk or think. They certainly are not persons in any of the normal ways that we tend to use the word to apply to ourselves or others.[15]

This is an especially important matter, for the issue concerning the care we ought to give to defective newborns is often framed in the language of rights—e.g., that children have a right to such care as a correlative of their right to life.[16] It remains questionable, however, whether moral rights can be attributed to newborns or very young children. For rights seem to require at a minimum that one be able to claim value for oneself, or able to exercise choice, or able to enter into contractual relations.[17] If this is the case, then the claim that newborns have a right to live that overrides all other claims or considerations is problematic.

3.1 Humanity and Suffering

However, even if "rights" language is hardly applicable to newborns, this does not mean that newborns have no value which provides a basis for their protection and care.[18] A newborn child is an earnest—the promissory note, if you will—of the goodness and vitality of our existence. Moreover, as humans, subject to the same fate and destiny, we have all learned that an essential aspect of our humanity is the opportunity we have to give special care to those particularly at the mercy of the human predicament. We learn little about the ethical presumption involved in the case of defective new-borns by asking if they are human persons. For the question is not whether they are human persons, but rather what kind of care we should give them in order for us to be humane.[19]

As G. J. Warnock observes, even though we do not regard infants as liable to judgments for their conduct on moral principles,

we do not for that reason regard them as morally insignificant, as having, that is, no moral *claims* upon rational beings. Why is this? Is it that they are in some sense, though not actual, yet potential beings, members, so to speak, of a potentially rational species? I do not think so. Infants no doubt could be said to be potentially rational; but is it for that reason that they are not to be, say physically maltreated? Not all imbeciles, I dare say, *are* potentially rational; but does it follow that, if they are reasonably judged to be incurable, they are then reasonably to be taken to have no moral claims? No: the basis of moral claims seems to me to be quite different. We may put it thus: just as a liability to be judged as a moral agent follows from one's general capability of alleviating, by moral action, the ills of the predicament, and is for that reason confined to rational beings, so the condition of being a proper 'beneficiary' of moral action is the capability of *suffering* the ills of the predicament—and for that reason is *not* confined to rational beings, nor even to potential members of that class. Things go badly, in general, if creatures suffer, better if they do not; to come within the ambit, then, of the ameliorative object of moral principles, is, not to be capable of contributing to such amelioration, but to be capable of suffering by its absence—that is capable of suffering.[20]

A similar argument has recently been made by Peter Singer as he contests the view that moral equality in any way depends on factual equality. For example the claim to equal treatment does not depend on IQ or any other measure since humans as individuals obviously differ in intelligence as well as almost all other abilities. In support of his position Peter Singer quotes Bentham's suggestion that:

It may one day come to be recognized that the number of the legs, the villosity of the skin, or the termination of the *os sacrum,* are reasons insufficient for abandoning a sensitive being to the same fate (fate of tyranny). What else is it that should trace the insuperable line? Is it the faculty of reason, or perhaps the faculty of discourse? But the fullgrown horse or dog is beyond comparison a more rational, as well as a more conversable animal, than an infant of a day, or a week, or even a month, old. But suppose they were otherwise, what would it avail? The question is not, Can they reason?, nor Can they talk?, but Can they suffer?

Singer thus argues that "if a being suffers, there can be no moral justification for refusing to take that suffering into consideration, and, indeed, to count it equally with the suffering of any other being."[21]

Such an argument does not claim that the life of defective newborns should be saved because human life is an absolute value. Rather it calls attention to our conviction that newborns, as suffering members of the human species, should be treated equal to others when it comes to life or death. We may decide that in certain circumstances life should not be preserved, but to do so amounts to deciding that all sufferers in similar circumstances, even ourselves, lose their lives.

This line of argument fails to detail the amount or kind of care we owe newborns. But it does articulate the moral basis for the responsibility we assume for the weak that come into the world as our children. Yet the question still remains whether some children are not disqualified from receiving the care we normally give to all children, precisely because they are defective. Does being defective constitute them as a class distinctively different from others who suffer? The question properly put, therefore, is not whether certain defects disqualify children as human, but rather whether these defects can materially alter the obligation we feel to care for them as fellow sufferers who also are our children.

The question seems to ask us to weigh the future capabilities of defective newborns to determine what quality care they should receive in the present. In effect we are suggesting that our responsibility to care for our children depends on their future potentiality. But surely this would apply also to so-called "normal" children, since we have good social indicators that children born in certain socioeconomic contexts have very poor potential. It becomes difficult to distinguish "normal" from "defective" children if the criterion is their future potential.

Perhaps we could differentiate between normal and defective newborn by the relative dependence each has on our medical technology. On this model some defective newborns would not be alive so much as an extension of certain technological procedures. In other words, we would *really* be dealing with dead children, "alive" only to the extent they are sustained by our medical technology. Such a strict criterion, however, exempts a defective newborn from the general observation that anyone's being alive includes the technological capacity of medicine to keep us alive.[22] It would seem arbitrary to exclude the defective newborn from those conditions of life we normally apply to all men.

In principle I see no reason why the defective newborn has any less claim to care than any newborn. In the language I have previously used, we should have moral care and respect for these children insofar as they suffer. For the crucial question that we should ask about these children is not whether they are less human because of their defects, but rather how we should act toward them in order that we do not arbitrarily cut them off from human community. In other words I see no reason why these children's defects materially disqualify them being regarded as children unless their defect is so severe there is little possibility that they will ever be able to respond to care.

Such a commitment falls short of determining, however, how much and what kind of care that we should be willing to give in order to sustain these children's lives. By a similar determination, moreover, it does not license our permitting (under certain conditions) them to die. It reminds us that we are dealing with suffering human beings who are not yet persons, but neither are they cabbages.

3.2 Parental Responsibility for Defective Newborns

The extent and kinds of care we should give newborns must be discussed in conjunction with the responsibilities we bear as parents. For these defective newborns are not just "newborns," or "suffering humans," they are children. In other words, what makes human birth human is partly our insistence that the infant is born into a role that carries expectations and duties embodied in the name, *child*.[23] Part of the tragedy of these cases may be that we live in a social situation where children are born devoid of the institutions to make them more than "newborns."

However, I suspect that many of these children are being allowed to die not because parents reject the role of being a parent but because they have a distorted notion of parental responsibility. Many parents seem to assume that they should be responsible to bring children into the world in a manner that can insure their happiness. Parents tend to think that they should not only be responsible for meeting their children's basic needs, but also must see that they do not have to suffer. Parental responsibility extends to assuring their children a happy and successful life.[24] Convictions like these reduce the options at birth to a perfect child or a dead child.

For example, there is a strong presumption behind the use of amniocentesis that we are obligated as parents to be responsible for our children's genetic characteristics in order to assure them a life free from suffering.[25] Yet this is an extraordinarily Promethean assumption about parenthood. A parenthood so freighted can bring little joy, for the responsibilities incumbent on the parent are simply overcoming. Moreover, it distorts child-rearing, as parents try to protect their children from the dangers and terrors of this world.

We can more fully explore the issues in the care of defective children the more critically we scrutinize the limits of our responsibilities as parents. We are certainly responsible to see that the basic physical, emotional and moral needs of our children are supplied. But I do not think that we can or should try to raise our children to insure their happiness.[26] We cannot and should not raise our children as if they could be protected against suffering and death. I suspect that the greatest injustice in some of these neonatal cases is done because we have lost sight of the fact that we must learn to love and care for our children as being destined for death. Our longing to protect our children from death has built neonatal units; yet the very presence of these units creates problems which remind us how we must learn again when it is time for our children to die. We should not under all conditions try to keep our children alive, but then neither should we kill some of our children because they do not conform to our ideal of "the good life."

4. Acting or Refraining

We can try to alleviate the dilemmas that we are facing in neonatal units by persuading ourselves that we are not really killing these children, but rather letting them die. We are "letting nature take its course." Part of the problem with this suggestion is it is no longer clear what "nature" means in such contexts, as nature has become an extension of our technology's ability to keep us alive. Certainly the idea that we are simply withholding treatment for some children is extremely questionable if we would have given the treatment to so-called "normal" children. If, for the "normal" child, "nature to take its course" means with the aid of all the technology we can muster, it can mean no less for the defective child.

Of course there is a wide range of cases where refraining from giving care produces no moral problem at all. For often care is withdrawn or not given simply because the prognosis is so poor that any care simply prolongs death rather than providing the means for life. Such a situation represents the paradigm for "letting someone die." Such judgments are left properly in the hands of doctors who have the skills to make such judgments.

In many cases, however, we seem to be withholding care not because we think the child will die, but because we are afraid it will live. In such cases it seems odd to suggest we are simply letting the child die by turning off the respirator or by refusing to perform the necessary surgery if "letting die" is properly only used to describe cases where we are no longer prolonging death. For we know that the child can only live with such care, and therefore a description of "letting die" seems strained.

For example, the withholding of normal life-giving surgery for a Down's child certainly means certain death. Yet rather than putting such children to death we make them wait out their time in order for us to say that we only "let them die." Surely in such cases there is little difference between withholding care and acting to put to death. It would seem more humane for us to inject an air bubble rather than making them wait out "nature's" course.

We continue to cling to the distinction between killing and letting die in such cases even though we intuitively feel that there is little difference between acting and refraining from giving care. On a theoretical level, moreover, it is clear that refraining is no less an "action" than an action, as it may in fact require greater consciousness than many of our so-called actions.[27] The question is not whether one acted or refrained from acting, but rather what is the proper description of the overall act.

The distinction between acting and refraining, I suspect, is really a misleading way of gesturing toward a more basic distinction whether what we owe to others is assistance or whether we can be content not to interfere.[28] We have an obligation, for example, not to kill others, but we do not necessarily have an obligation to keep someone alive by rendering aid.[29] Our positive duties are dependent on the establishment of relationships that make intelligible our further responsibilities. For example, we normally think that we do have duties to aid our children beyond our obligations to strangers. To employ the language of refraining to "solve" these neonatal dilemmas amounts then to transforming our duty toward our children into the duty we acknowledge to a stranger—namely, noninterference.

4.1 Roles and Responsibilities

We are drawn to the idea that we are simply refraining to give care because we are concerned to describe our action in a manner congruent with our assumed roles and identity. As John Casey suggests, "The view we take of a man's character, or of his role in a certain type of situation, sets limits not only on what we can regard him as responsible for in that situation but also on what we can properly describe him as doing or refraining from doing."[30] The roles that constitute our lives are in fact complex patterns of expectations that others learn to rely on. These expectations provide the context for attribution of responsibility, praise, and blame. Often we are praised or blamed for actions that we never said that we would or would not do explicitly, because the actions are simply embodied in the role that we have assumed and for which we reap advantages and disadvantages. The distinction between acting and refraining, in the context of neonatal dilemmas, is an attempt to defeat certain ascriptions of responsibility for two extremely significant roles: parents and doctors.

We normally assume the parental role involves caring for our children; at a minimum this would seem to involve the responsibility to see to their physical well-being. Hence we would hold responsible parents who neglected their child to the extent of the child dying of malnutrition. We *could* describe the cause of death as a lack of food, or that they refrained from giving her food.

Yet we cannot help but feel that such descriptions of the case would be extremely misleading as moral descriptions (though it might well assign the proximate cause of death in appropriate medical terms). Given our normal expectations of how parents should behave, however, we feel it appropriate to say that this child died of parental neglect—in fact they put her to death.

I suspect what is at stake in the cases occurring in neonatal units and the reason we use acting-refraining language is that we are not sure if it is a proper expectation to ask parents to use all the medical technology available in order to keep their children alive. The acting-refraining distinction allows us to mark these off as special cases in a way that does not defeat our normal assumptions that parents should care for the physical well-being of their children—i.e., there are limits to the positive aid that parents are expected to give to keep their children alive.

However, would we not be morally more healthy if we described these cases for what they often are—namely, putting these children to death because there are limits to what we can ask parents to do for the preservation of children? To continue to use the acting-refraining distinction lets us off the hook, and as a result we learn nothing about what we take the role of parenting to be. I suspect our social system may be willing to let parents kill their children much earlier and for reasons we may feel are less than justified, but at least by stating the issue clearly we have a better idea of what we are involved in. Only when we rightly describe what we are doing can we begin to develop necessary safeguards. For example, it may be necessary for doctors to have some protection from parents who may well have the legal right to ask doctors to withdraw therapy from their children before the doctor thinks it medically justified.[31]

It must be admitted, however, that doctors have had an equal stake in seeing the distinction between acting and refraining maintained. Doctors are pledged to protect and care for life. One of the cardinal principles of medicine states that the doctor should never directly take life or intervene to hasten death. The doctor's role is to cherish and protect life. Doctors guard this jealously precisely because they know how intimately the power to continue life is linked with the ability to end it.

The distinction between acting and refraining allows doctors to continue the illusion that in the neonatal cases with which we are concerned they continue to be concerned primarily with the care of life. Our assumption that we are refraining to act allows us to keep our role expectations intact so that other people can continue to count on doctors for life-enhancing therapy. The importance of this for the practice of medicine in a pluralist society cannot be ignored; society demands an absolutist ethic of doctors for the protection of life, not because it trusts doctors but because it does not. We fear the possibility that doctors might become captive of one group's sense of what counts for life in a manner that renders our own existence problematic. A doctor's commitment to care first for a patient's physical well-being monitors the fear that some would have him deny the physical life of others due to the "quality" of their life.

4.2   Caring and Curing

I suspect part of the problem that doctors face when confronted by these kinds of cases stems from the assumption by doctors and patients alike that the care (the doctor brings) must be synonymous with cure. For many doctors a patient is medically dead when you can no longer cure.[32] This attitude becomes especially pernicious when cure is correlated with an idea of health that promises general well-being rather than minimal physical function. This broadened sense of health opens medicine for use for non-medical ends. There is a great deal of difference, certainly, between breast enlargement and the use of doctors for torture, but each assumes that medicine can and should be used for ends not having to do with a patient's physical health. Some of the children we are letting die for "medical reasons" are in fact victims of this expanded meaning of health.[33]

The medicinal role does not get its justification or goal from making people happy. The securing of health often does not relieve suffering, but only continues suffering. The care the doctor is required to give is not a care that can provide happiness. His task is not to make a family secure or to protect parents from the suffering occasioned by a retarded child. The doctor's task is to secure the health of such children, for they are his patients, even though it may mean tragedy for a family.

Of course someone should be concerned about the effects on the family. I am simply suggesting that such concerns should not enter into the doctor's calculation of his responsibility. One of the marks of a morally healthy society is its ability to differentiate roles and tasks for the care of its members. Medicine as a moral art is dependent on such differentiation of function to create the forms and limits of the care doctors should provide. We must not forget that medicine more than any other function today is close to priestcraft, as it holds the power over life and death. (The church has surely been right to restrict and control its priests who also happen to be doctors, as such a person combines what are perhaps the two most powerful roles men can obtain.) Such power is rightfully limited by the doctor's concern to cure patients, not diseases, to secure the health of this patient, not mankind, and to provide physical health, not personal well-being. The doctor can limit his care—for medicine is the moral art of knowing how to care for the sufferer—*only if he has the assurance that there are other kinds of care present in the community.*

Yet there are signs that we do not exist in a society that provides the range of care necessary for the preservation of humane communities. This is amply illustrated in the cases we are discussing, as it is clear that doctors can no longer know what kind of assumptions underlie parenthood. Doctors have tried to substitute further medical skill for the breakdown of community that should direct that skill. Such a substitution, however, cannot be successful, for it is simply not clear how or if it is possible to practice medicine as a moral art in a society of strangers. At least doctors must be willing to force their patients to understand the limits of medicine. The consumers of medicine must be forced to see that medicine is not the technologically neutral science to be bought by the highest bidder, but one of the ways we as a community learn to care for one another as beings destined to death.

If we had this kind of moral community then it might be possible for doctors to care for some children without subjecting them to a mercy grown overwhelming by technology. For the care that is the moral art of the doctor does not mean that every child should be subjected to every technique available to keep it alive. Care is not synonomous with manipulation. As Ramsey says, "there comes a time when to cherish and respect life means to care but *only* to care for the dying, no longer to oppose death, to accept its coming, to comfort and to keep company with the dying, not to prolong their dying but to make human presence in that solitude, never to desert them, to insure as much dignity as possible to the dying in their passage."[34] What we must admit is that some children are born with death as close as their next breath. The great art of medicine is to care for them even when you cannot cure them.

The problem is that we live in a moral context when doctors and patients have both conspired to deny that medicine is no cure for death. I suspect that we will get no help on these difficult decisions in neonatal units until parents and doctors are willing to talk realistically of what should be the limits of human care.

5. Conclusion

I have no doubt that for many this paper ends with a whimper rather than a bang. For it may be felt that I have offered little help for those who have to deal on a day-to-day basis with the kind of dilemma *Time* describes as "The Hardest Choice." (Cases for ethicists are always "interesting," but for doctors they are matters about which they have to make a decision.) I have tried, however, to sketch a framework within which ethical reflection must proceed, if we are to learn better how to deal with these children. It may be helpful if I summarize what I take that framework to be.

The fundamental issue that provides the background for the kind and amount of care defective newborns should receive is the obligations of parents to care for their children. Because parents naturally want to care for their children, we often forget that such care is also a moral expectation. The defective newborn challenges us to articulate these "natural" assumptions, however, for it is not clear whether we should "normally" expect parental care to aid their children under all conditions.

I have argued, nevertheless, that parents *do* have a positive obligation to care for their children. Children are not the property of parents to dispose of as they wish.[35] How far does this parental obligation reach, however, when it comes to parents' duty to secure the child's physical integrity by means offered by medicine? The amount of care should not be determined by the extent of the child's "defect," unless that defect is so physiologically severe that there is no potential for the child ever to benefit or respond to human care.

Furthermore, it is not clear whether the state should attempt legally to embody parental obligation in these cases. The state has an interest in requiring parents to meet the basic obligations they have to their children; yet it is a matter of debate whether such care is a "basic" obligation.

In the absence of legal and moral consensus the doctor is put in a precarious position. What has been revealed is how dependent our medicine is on its underlying moral communities, such as the family, to give it moral direction. But it may be difficult for doctors to prevent themselves from becoming the agents of death for couples who no longer view their newborns as children.

I would recommend at the least that each hospital and doctor begin to draw up a statement of procedures concerning the care of defective newborns. This should be given to couples as early as possible so they might have an opportunity to find other institutions or doctors whose policies conform more exactly with their own. (I recognize there is the added problem of the mother who only comes to the doctor when she is in labor. This is particularly important as it is just such a mother who is most likely to have trouble.) Developing such statements would not resolve the problems we are facing in this area, but the effect would help us begin the kind of public discussion that must take place if we are to find ways to treat these children humanly in a manner that respects them and preserves our own dignity as well as that of our communities.

14. Medicine as a Tragic Profession

Hegel spoke of tragedy as "the conflict of right with right"; what makes any protagonist's situation tragic is that he inevitably has to choose between wrong and wrong. It is with this in mind that I have spoken of the physician's moral dilemmas as tragic. The moral resources of his culture, of our own culture, offer no solution for him. What matters most in a period in which human life is tragic is to have the strength to resist false solutions. The characteristic temptation of the modern world is utilitarianism. For utilitarianism in all its versions aspires to provide a criterion, a way of judging between rival and conflicting goods to maximize utility. But the goods and the rights which define our contemporary conflicts are incommensurable. There is no higher criterion. There is no neutral concept of utility.

The medical profession ought not therefore to look for solutions to philosophical theorizing; what philosophy has to tell them is precisely why they cannot hope for solutions. For a philosopher to try to go beyond this would be for him to misunderstand either the present situation or the scope and limits of his discipline. A philosopher offering positive moral advice in this situation would be a comic character introduced into a tragedy: Imagine Socrates introducing himself with advice for Antigone or Creon, or Plato trying to counsel Philoctetes, Neoptolemus and Odysseus. Yet to understand even this is perhaps to transform the perspective in which moral problems of medicine are viewed; and such a transformation can only be effected by philosophy.[1]

1. Medicine as a Moral Art

It has become a commonplace for those working in medical ethics to claim that medicine is a moral art. However, like most commonplace assumptions it is not very clear what such a claim means or entails. Usually it is used to emphasize that medicine is not a neutral technology manned by impersonal robots. But on analysis medicine seems to involve a complex interrelation of moral convictions and technological skill that is difficult to characterize.[2]

Of course medicine obviously involves moral issues in respect to such matters as death and dying, experimentation, abortion, to name just a few. But to associate the "morality" of medicine with its involvement with explicit moral concerns misses the force of the claim that medicine is a moral art. For the claim is not just that medicine involves matters of moral concern, but that the very practice of medicine entails moral convictions that shape its fundamental nature.

The emphasis on the moral presuppositions necessarily entailed in the meaning of health, disease, and illness thus seems to be closer to carrying the force of the claim that medicine is a moral art.[3] But while it is clear that our understanding of disease involves matters that are extra-medical, it is not clear exactly how "moral" convictions are crucial to our understanding of disease and illness. It may be, as Illich suggests, that "culture and health coincide," but that does not mean we can conclude that all designation of disease is normative in a moral sense.[4]

Finally, the claim that medicine is a moral art is used by some to emphasize medicine's commitment to care for other humans. This emphasis has found its most forceful expression in the work of Paul Ramsey, who argues that medicine embodies in a particularly intense form our general moral commitment to one another. It is Ramsey's view that medicine already embodies an appropriate ethic for its task—the canon of loyalty between the physician and his patient—and the only problem is whether that commitment can withstand the utilitarian-inspired assault of the research imperative. Ramsey's concern, therefore, is whether our civilization has a sufficient public ethos to support the central ethical commitments of medicine.[5]

While I have some sympathy with Ramsey's position in this respect, I think that his concentration on the "canon of loyalty" between the physician and patient oversimplifies the kinds of moral commitment that the practice of medicine entails. First it oversimplifies the commitment of the physician to his patient, as the question is seldom *whether* the physician should be loyal to the patient but *how?* Second, the "canon of loyalty" does not provide an adequate moral expression for public medicine as an institution. And finally, the "canon of loyalty" does not help us understand what kind of moral commitments we must make as a society in order to have a patient-centered medicine.

Indeed, in terms of this last problem Ramsey's position tends to lead us to think that what medicine needs is more support from a libertarian ethic that supports the freedom and rights of the individual. But, as I hope to show, such an ethic is not sufficient to support the kind of ethos necessary to sustain the kind of profession and care that medicine should involve.

In the hope of throwing some light on the physician's commitment to the patient, it is my contention that we need to direct our attention to MacIntyre's suggestion that medicine involves tragedy. The tragic nature of medicine is not rooted only in dilemmas unique to our time, but is constitutive of the profession of medicine as a practice. In sum, my contention is that medicine is a moral art because it must be guided by convictions that sustain the effort to care in the face of death. Indeed, it is exactly part of the crisis of modern medicine, so aptly described by MacIntyre, that the convictions necessary for such a task seem to be absent.

I have three interests that I hope will be served by shifting the analysis to the question of the tragic nature of medical care. First, it is a way of trying to raise some perennial issues involved in the practice of medicine. It is often asserted that the moral problems associated with medicine are more pressing today because of the development of scientifically and technologically sophisticated medical therapies. However, I hope to show that the emphasis on the moral problems occasioned by medical technology has failed to denote the moral concerns that have been and must be present when one person seeks to heal and care for another. From this perspective I think we will be able to see that the moral crisis in contemporary medicine is not the result of the development of scientific medicine, but our failure to have a sufficient sense of the physical and moral limits involved in any attempt to help and care for one another.

Second, medicine as a tragic profession suggests that medical ethics cannot be limited to casuistical analysis of particular sets of problems and issues. Rather, the moral concerns that are basic involve the character of the physician, patient, and the community that sustains them. Discussions of medical ethics must, therefore, involve issues of political philosophy and in particular the status of special relations in a society.

In this respect I hope to show that genuine progress has been made in recent work in medical ethics, but it is not of the kind that many have anticipated. For example, we are not any closer to determining what kind of care we should give to defective newborns. But I think we have come to a better understanding of what kind of activity medicine is and the kind of ethos required to sustain it. For, odd as it may sound, our greatest difficulty in developing "medical ethics" has been to know how to describe what kind of activity medicine involves. At the same time, however, I think our understanding of medicine as a moral art has challenged the dominant paradigm of contemporary ethical theory. For we have come to see that the moral commitments made in medicine cannot be adequately expressed in "principles," but involve convictions that require narrative display.[6]

Finally, I think the emphasis on medicine as a tragic profession helps denote the continuity between the kind of issues raised by medicine and the rest of our lives. Medicine is an important area for moral reflection because there we have raised with particular cogency questions no moral man can avoid. "Medical ethics" is neither a unique form of moral reflection or applied ethics, but rather a significant form of human activity that helps us to chart our way in other aspects of our lives.

1.1 Statement of the Problem

Of course, the assertion that medicine is a tragic profession begs all the issues—what do we mean by tragic? In what sense is medicine tragic? What does a profession involve? And even more puzzling, what would it mean to understand oneself to be a practitioner of a tragic profession? In order to begin to make headway on these questions I think it is instructive to look briefly at Illich's attack on modern medicine. For it seems to me that Illich has mistakenly assumed that the development of modern medicine necessarily must exclude a sense of the tragic. His concern for a proper appreciation of the latter has thus led him to assume that we would be better off without the medical care we currently, in Illich's view, suffer from.

Illich argues that modern medicine is literally dangerous to our health. He bases his argument on the incidence of iatrogenic illness in order to show that our professional and physician-based health care system makes us sick for three reasons: "It must produce clinical damage that outweighs its potential benefits; it cannot but enhance even as it obscures the political conditions that render society unhealthy; and it tends to mystify and to expropriate the power of the individual to heal himself and to shape his environment."[7] This medical epidemic has been made worse by the loss of the sense that medicine is a moral enterprise. Thus what was formerly "considered an abuse of confidence and a moral fault can now be rationalized into the occasional breakdown of equipment and operators."[8]

Medicine according to Illich has become the paradigmatic form of oppression of a technological society, namely, it is self-imposed oppression that is not noticed as such because it is assumed that we benefit from it. In an argument reminiscent of Jacques Ellul, Illich suggests that there is no medical remedy for medical nemesis, there is no technological way to control technology, but rather the only solution is for the laity to recover the will to care for themselves. In Illich's terms we can no longer let the medical enterprise sap "the will of people to suffer their reality," but we can seize control only by our willingness to see suffering as "an inevitable part of our conscious coping with reality."[9]

Generally, I suspect that most of us respond to Illich according to our current physical condition. If we feel extraordinarily healthy, I suspect we think, "by God that is right." If we are a little under the weather, we may think that there is a lot to what Illich says, we surely are an overmedicalized society, but we are still glad that we have a few doctors out there. If we are really feeling bad, we tend to discount Illich as rubbish and thank God that we have this nice hospital in which we can receive the attention we think we deserve.

Of course, these kinds of response fail to do justice to the strengths or weaknesses of Illich's arguments. However, they do help illustrate, I think, that Illich's target is not really modern medicine as such but rather the presumptuous claims with which physician and patient alike mistakenly endow modern medicine. Such presumptuous attitudes, however, can as easily be associated with the past forms of medicine as with the scientific form practiced by our society.

Because Illich confuses the ideology or theory of medicine with its practice,[10] those who criticize Illich often do so in a way that misses the force of his position. For example, Lewis Thomas is certainly correct that Illich has not shown statistically that we suffer more from doctor-caused illness than we would if such medical care were not available.[11] Indeed, it is not clear how anyone could show that more good than evil results from modern medicine. Because Illich has put the matter in this way he seems to be making us choose between having modern medicine or none at all. Since it is not clear what Illich's alternative would be, I think most of us, no matter how sympathetic we may be with aspects of Illich's argument, would continue to choose modern medicine.

But that is simply a false issue. The issue is not whether we must choose between having medicine or having none, but rather the issue is what kind of limits should we accept, not as arbitrary impositions, but as appropriate forms that define the nature of our existence and, consequently, the nature of our medical care. Illich challenges us to embody a story which can sustain medical care in the face of a recurrent dilemma: what we are able to do will not suffice and may even make things worse. For in spite of claims to the contrary, we surely continue to assume that it is the doctor's duty to preserve life even when health cannot be restored, and even when the preservation of life means we must exist in pain and suffering.

Ernest Becker has pointed out that modern science, with the death of God, has to assume the role of supplying a theodicy to sustain us in the face of our obvious deaths.[12] In that spirit Lewis Thomas, in response to Illich, argues that medicine has just begun to reach the status of science. And that now "the way is open to science, and this is the great point missed by Illich. Having proved, once and for all, that science can provide conclusive measures for disease control, we have begun to discern clues, feasible scientific approaches to each of the major diseases still at large."[13] But that is exactly the presumption with which Illich is at war—namely, that medicine holds out the prospect of the eradication of pain, suffering, and death—for such a presumption, according to Illich, will destroy us.

In fairness to Thomas, however, it should be pointed out that he agrees that "perhaps there will always be, as Illich maintains, human problems that are not the business of medicine, in which we are likely to do more harm than good by meddling. Unhappiness, discontent, anomie, worry about meaning, ill will, grabbiness, and the loss of nerve are huge problems for our society but they are not medical problems. Medicine's professional task is the prevention and cure of illness, most of all the prevention of premature death.''[14] But such a response begs the issue, since Illich's question is what should count for illness and/or premature death; and equally important, what should be the convictions that guide doctor and patient alike in knowing how to respond to them.

1.2 Development of the Issue

In the rest of this essay I will try to show how Illich has failed to see that the practice of modern medicine is, in spite of some claims to the contrary, a tragic profession. I will do this by looking at what it means for medicine to be a profession and the inherit limits of judgment in medicine. By developing this latter theme I hope to show how Thomas' trust in science is a philosophical mistake, as the inherent particularity of medical judgment necessarily cannot avoid error. In the process I will try to suggest that the lack of moral consensus to guide medical care in our society intensifies its tragic character.

2. The Profession of Medicine

It is not my intention to try to provide a satisfactory analysis of what a profession is.[15] Rather, I will simply propose a relatively noncontroversial list of attributes that I think can be used to characterize medicine as a profession. This is not to deny that there may be powerful arguments that we would be better off if medicine were not given the autonomy of a profession. For example, some suggest that the deprofessionalization of medicine would make us take more responsibility for our health as well as more nearly institutionalize the appropriate limits of medicine as an art. However, I think it best to begin with our current sense of medicine as a profession in order to better appreciate in what ways it may peculiarly be so.

There are five primary characteristics that help us understand in what sense medicine is a profession:

(1) Those engaged in medicine do so "for a living" rather than "for fun." In other words doctors are not amateurs and/or dilettantes, but rather are committed to developing a high level of expertise as a life-task. I take it that it is in this sense that a doctor and some athletes can be thought of as "professionals."[16]

(2) There is a recognized body of skills or knowledge that one must become familiar with through training and apprenticeship. Moreover, there are some who act as custodians of those skills by enforc-

ing criteria of certification on those who wish to enter the profession.

(3) A profession is both an economic monopoly and largely self-regulating and this state of affairs is given statutory status by the society. In order to be a profession the society must officially find ways to institutionalize its trust in the profession's self-regulation both by policing the requisite knowledge, and by enforcing an internal ethic appropriate to its activity.

(4) "The professions are almost always involved with matters which from time to time are among the greatest personal concerns that humans have; physical health, psychic well-being, liberty, and the like."[17] As a result, the professions morally reflect the basic goods that are thought to be necessary for life in that society.

(5) Finally, "the professions almost always involve at their core a significant interpersonal relationship between the professional on one hand, and the person who is thought to require the professional's services: the patient or the client."[18]

In this section I will primarily be dealing with characteristics 3, 4, and 5. I will be trying to show the basic moral convictions that chart medicine as a profession and how they are frequently incompatible.[19] But more to the point I will argue that the tragic nature of medicine does not just involve conflicts of value, but the role limitations that must be part of the doctor's self-understanding. In the next section I will deal with the characteristics in 1 and 2, as I will try to demonstrate how the "expertise" of skill and knowledge inherent to medicine necessarily results in tragic error.

By calling medicine a tragic profession I am suggesting that it reflects the limits of our existence.[20] These limits are often manifest in the conflicting claims upon us, in our necessary faithfulness to parochial but nonetheless overriding obligations, in our self-made disasters and errors, and often in our helplessness. Of course, disasters, errors, and helplessness are not necessarily tragic, but they often become such when they are involved in our attempt to care for one another. Tragedy is not helplessness, but our helplessness may be a manifestation of the tragic as it reminds us of our finitude.

Nor do I wish to suggest that medicine is somehow more tragic than other aspects of our lives. However, due to medicine's involvement with the basic movements of our lives—birth, growth, sex, death—its practice both manifests and embodies more intensely the tragic nature of our existence. Because medicine so readily makes us conscious of the tragic, we have ironically tried to use it as a means to deny the tragic. But as I will try to show, this self-deception has only intensified the tragic nature of medicine by making us less able to subject medicine to its proper office for our lives. Medicine is not more tragic than other aspects of our lives, but if it fails to be formed by a proper sense of the tragic its potential for moral destructiveness is increased.

2.1 The Conflict of Value and the Profession of Medicine

It is clear from the above characteristics that a profession involves an internalized code of ethics that may or may not be formalized. It is generally assumed that such codes are consistent within themselves. However, as has been recently demonstrated in the field of law, the lawyer's commitment to his client often conflicts with his responsibilities as an officer of the court.[21] Steven Toulmin, relying on Freedman's analysis, has argued that such conflicts are also present in the practice of medicine.

According to Toulmin, part of the conflict is the result of the modern "alliance between medical practice and science, which has put the profession's priorities in question, and introduced ambiguities into the public's perception of medicine and the physician. For how do doctors who are also involved in—or with—the activity of scientific research determine the relative urgency of the professional claims facing them, on the one hand as physicians, on the other hand as scientists?"[22] Of course, it can be suggested that while this may in fact be a conflict for some it is not a conflict in principle since it is clear that the physician must always give priority to the patient's welfare.

However, this response may be too shallow in that it fails to appreciate how deeply patient or clinical medicine is interdependent with research medicine today. Even if that is the case, however, it can be pointed out that the requirement of informed consent still stands as a check against the research imperative in medicine. Yet as Toulmin points out, there is a real question whether the distinction between "free and informed" and "coerced" consent is powerful enough to deal with these matters. "It has frequently been argued, for instance, that any prison is an 'inherently coercive environment,' so that consent by prisoners to participate in human experimentation is always of questionable force. Taken on its own terms, this is an impressive argument; but, in return, we might ask whether *sickness itself* is not also 'inherently coercive'; and whether, in virtue of the natural authority a physician exercises toward anyone in that condition, the patient will not inevitably feel constrained to participate as a research subject for any scientific project in which he perceives 'his' doctor as having an interest. That argument provides both sufficient grounds for public anxiety over the current close alliance between medical practice and biomedical research, *and also* reasons to re-examine with care the institutional relations between—particularly, the traditional buffers between—the work of the physician and that of the scientist."[23]

While I think it is clear that Toulmin has located a problem of potential conflict of value there are other sorts of conflict that are more pressing in the practice of normal, nonresearch medicine. In various ways it is assumed that the physician has an overriding commitment to care for the patient—in Ramsey's phrase, the patient must be treated as a person. Lester King has put this well as he suggested that "the physician enters into a special relationship with a patient as a person, a relationship that involves marked circumscription of context. The physician and the patient form a relatively isolated system, in which the physician as healer tries to cure the patient. All else is irrelevant."[24]

However, on analysis this emphasis on the physician's commitment to the individual patient tends to obscure other, quite legitimate duties the doctor has. For example the doctor has duties "toward the public health authorities, or, where relevant, toward the institution within which he practices—clinic, hospital, university, or group practices—and even, in the case of an industrial, prison, or other institutional clinic, toward the organization within which it is located."[25]

To make the commitment to the patient the primary basis for the doctor's moral task simply fails to do justice to the reality of medicine as a social system. As Jonsen and Hellegers have pointed out,

> Medicine has, in recent years, evolved from a practice, a private technical interaction between two parties, through a profession, a socially coherent, publicly recognized group that defines the conditions under which those private transactions take place to an institution. By an institution, we mean a complex interaction of professional, paraprofessionals, and the public, at informational economic and occupational levels, in identifiable physical environment, whose coordinated decisions and action have magnified public impact and is recognized culturally and legally as affecting the public welfare in a significant way . . . Modern medicine, then, is an institution that incorporates a profession that practices a technique and an art.[26]

As such, medicine reaches far beyond the care of the individual patient and, at least according to Jonsen and Hellegers, requires a sense of the common good to give it moral direction. But obviously the common good may well conflict at times with the good of the individual patient.

However, more important for the thesis of this paper is the recognition that the doctor has not one, but several parallel obligations to a single patient that may conflict. For example it may be that in order to treat a patient adequately the doctor has to violate the rule of confidentiality. The patient, however, may refuse to have his privacy violated and the duty of confidentiality may prevent the physician from giving the patient the treatment he needs. Nor is it always clear that the physician by following his own commitment to the patient is doing what the patient feels is in his best interest. Reflection on those physicians trying to prevent Gary Gilmore's dying in order to save him for the firing squad is but a dramatic example of a necessary conflict in medicine.

We tend to think of situations like these as conflicts, but the doctor may assume that his overriding commitment to the preservation of human life means that from his point of view no conflict is present. But we are becoming increasingly aware that this kind of rule, like all rules, requires interpretation. In the past the interpretation of such a rule could be entrusted to the doctor and patient. The doctor was assumed to have authority for interpretation, not because of his technical skill, but because he represented the community's wisdom about conditions necessary for a worthwhile life, the responsibilities of parents, etc. To be sure, their convictions varied from place to place, family to family, and individual to individual, but the differences were the nuances of a theme. The patient could expect the doctor to *tell* what *he* thought was necessary, not just to spell out alternatives, because the doctor and patient were bound together in a network of trust secured by common expectations. Moreover, each was sustained by a community that understood that such judgments could result in error even though everyone had done his best.

But in a society of strangers it is crucial to make the meaning and application of rules independent of interpretation. Rules must be applied impersonally and uniformly in order to avoid the arbitrariness we assume must be part of all "judgments." The necessity to impose rules uniformly, however, often occasions disastrous results. Thus, where at one time the doctor and patient simply knew when the time had come to die, we are forced today to keep many alive beyond all reason. As MacIntyre suggests, "the physician now finds himself in a tragic dilemma. Consider the case of recently born crippled infants where heroic efforts may preserve *either* a needless bundle of distorted and suffering nerves and tissues *or*—sometimes against all probable calculations—a human child, physically imperfect but with real potential, perhaps even a Helen Keller. Any rule which relieves the physician of the burden of extending suffering uselessly imposes on him the burden of taking innocent life wantonly; and no rule would be worst of all."[27] Whatever the status of the rule for preserving life may be, it clearly is not a rule designed to free the doctor from tragedy.

2.2 Moral Limits of Role Differentiation

These last issues, however, raise what I take to be a more difficult problem involved in the moral charter of medicine as a profession. As I noted above, it is one of the presuppositions of a profession that there is a special and privileged relationship between the professional and the patient. Each of the parties in the relationship is involved in role-differentiated behavior. "This is significant because it is the nature of role-differentiated behavior that it often makes it both appropriate and desirable for the person in a particular role to put to one side considerations—that would otherwise be relevant if not decisive."[28] In other words, role-differentiated behavior often alters or eliminates certain moral considerations that would obtain if it were not for the existence of that role.

The paradigmatic form of this behavior is that between a parent and a child. In almost all contexts and social situations we think parents are entitled, if not obligated, to prefer the interests of their own children over those of others. "That is to say, it is regarded as appropriate for a parent to allocate excessive goods to his or her own children, even though other children may have substantially more pressing and genuine needs for these same items. If one were trying to decide what the right way was to distribute assets among a group of children all of whom were strangers to oneself, the relevant moral considerations would be very different from those that would be thought to obtain once one's own children were in the picture. In the role of a parent, the claims of other children vis-a-vis one's own are, if not rendered morally irrelevant, certainly rendered less morally significant."[29]

To be in a profession is to be enmeshed in role-differentiated behavior of this sort. This means that the role of the professional is to prefer in a variety of ways the interests of the client or patient over those of individuals generally. It is assumed that the physician is justified in bracketing all other moral judgments that might be relevant because the role of the physician and the services associated with it are good in themselves. In other words, it is assumed that the doctor's willingness to block out all other concerns apart from those of how to care for his patient is justified because we think the institution of medicine in itself is morally a good thing.

Yet we cannot ignore the fact that we pay high costs in order to allow for this kind of "professionalization." Some of these costs are not intrinsically linked to the roles, but their accidental form does not make them any less real. In this respect I am thinking of how such roles often justify or encourage a patronizing behavior, unjustified paternalism, as well as a dangerous inequity of power between the professional and the patient. Or worse the moral status of such roles can be used to justify moral irresponsibility by declaring ourselves as morally incompetent in all other nonprofessional contexts. Moreover, the professional is tempted to relate to only those aspects of the person that his services are meant to deal with. This becomes particularly destructive for the professional inasmuch as too often the professional role becomes one's dominant role—we become our profession.

However, as I noted, these are costs that are not inherent to the role-differentiated behavior characteristic of a profession and in particular of medicine. It does, however, indicate the special care that should be taken in the selection and training of those who take up those professions. They should have the character to be able to withstand the subtle and unavoidable temptations of being a "professional."

More relevant to our purposes is the cost such role-differentiated behavior exacts of society itself. For society must be willing to have its own general goods threatened in order to have doctors perform their tasks—murderers must be healed, some cared for who will not contribute to the general good, and energy and resources drained off into the fight to save those that are already beyond their ability to participate in our social order.

I am not suggesting that we should not be willing to pay these costs; indeed, I think that we should. Rather I am trying to remind us that just as successful medical therapy does not bring happiness to the individual, so also the successful operation of medicine as an institution of society does not bring societal happiness. Yet we as a society think that the goods served by medicine are so basic they justify letting the doctor be free from those wider moral issues.

But this means we must be clear that medicine's moral task necessarily involves a sense of the tragic. For the doctor to assume overriding loyalty to his or her patient may well entail tragic results for others and perhaps even for that patient. A parent's obligation to his or her children may have tragic implications but does not mean that such claims are voided. The same is also true of the doctor's obligations. What is needed is not a change in the moral commitment, but a story and community that help sustain those kinds of commitments.

2.3 Authority and the Professions

We no longer live in the social order that provided the moral presuppositions to sustain the differentiation of role required by the professions. The presupposition of the practice of medicine as role-differentiated behavior was the existence of a shared and socially established morality. I am not suggesting that in the past medicine was personal as opposed to the impersonality of technological medicine. In the past, doctor and patient may have been "strangers," but they still were bound together by their tradition which set their expectations. That is, "the physician could assume that the patient's attitudes towards life and death would be roughly the same as his own, and vice versa. Hence the patient in putting him or herself into the hands of his or her physician could feel that he or she was not relinquishing his or her moral autonomy."[30]

The patients could "trust" their physician, not because of a "personal" relation, but because it was assumed that they shared the same values and beliefs. It was assumed that the doctor was an authority to be trusted, not just because of his knowledge, but because he represented moral convictions commonly shared. Our societies could entrust the development of certain goods, e.g., education to teachers, health to the medical profession, because it assumed that a moral division of labor was the best way of allowing the manifold goods of our culture to flourish.

But as MacIntyre has argued, we no longer live in a society that has a shared moral tradition. Rather, we exist as a social order that embodies fragments of past moral convictions that are simply incommensurable. As a result we no longer exist as friends, but morally the demand for autonomy requires us to meet one another only as strangers.[31]

In such a moral order the idea of authority always appears as a threat to my autonomy. As a result, the idea of a profession becomes anomalous—it is not quite a craftsman's guild, not quite a trade union, not quite anything. The profession's characteristics have lost their connection with the principles which, in their variety, made a relatively unified whole. This is what has happened in our culture and it at once makes the profession's peculiar claims to authority, and the kind of role-differentiated behavior dependent on that, morally unintelligible.[32] Yet paradoxically, this lacuna also increases the demand for professional probity as the profession claims "autonomy" in an attempt to secure itself from the chaotic general ethos.

But if this is the case it also means that our reliance on the professional may have tragic results. Even when a community of moral beliefs is lacking, "trust between strangers becomes much more questionable than when we can safely assume such a community. Nobody can rely on anyone else's judgments on his or her behalf until he or she knows what the other person believes. It follows that nobody can accept the moral authority of another in virtue simply of his professional position. We are thrust back by our social condition into a form of moral autonomy. Individualistic moral philosophers have portrayed autonomy as a central moral good. In the perspective of the above it is rather a situation of the last resort."[33]

I have tried to suggest above that it takes a set of very substantive convictions for a society to give power to the profession of medicine as a tragic profession—that is, as a profession that cares when it cannot cure. However, that tragedy is only increased when the profession is left without the accompanying societal convictions. For then medicine is in the danger of being grasped by another set of convictions that promises more than it can ever deliver, namely, the attempt to insure autonomy as an end in itself.

Yet when the moral commitments of medicine are formed by the story of the autonomous individual it requires the eradication of tragedy. For the demands of autonomy require that medicine, and all other "helping professions,'' free us from our natural and self-made fates. But as we shall see in the next section that is exactly what medicine is not capable of doing. Ironically, because we have failed to account for medicine's tragic character we have, as Illich suggests, become far too subject to it. Medicine's attempt to insure us against fate has led us to call our dependence on it the quest for freedom.

3. Judgment and Error in Medicine

I noted above that the claim that medicine is a profession entails not only a standard of behavior but also a field of skills and knowledge that the practitioner must learn to use. In most treatments of medical ethics this aspect is ignored because it is generally assumed to be subsumed by the question of certification. In other words, the only question is one of responsibility—does he or she know what any good doctor should know for the proper treatment of their patients?

However, I want to argue that the matter is much more complex than this, as the very nature of the kind of knowledge and skill practiced by the doctor necessarily involves error. Error in medicine is not just the result of bad judgment or malfeasance, but, as MacIntyre and Gorovitz have argued, results from the very nature of how explanation and prediction work in medical diagnosis.[34]

It is generally assumed that in medical science, like so-called ''pure'' or ''hard'' science, mistakes are due either to the limitations of the present state of natural science, i.e., ignorance, or to the negligence or ineptitude of the scientist. Gorovitz and MacIntyre observe that this view of error is correlative of the scientist's view that he is dealing with universals and relations between universals. Thus, ''the scientist looks for law-like relationships between properties; particulars occur in this account only as the bearers of properties, and the implied concept of a particular is of a contingent collection of properties. To explain the behavior of a particular is nothing else than to subsume its particular properties under the relevant law-like generalization; to predict is to use the same stock of law-like generalization about the relevant properties. Notice that on this view predictive failure in science can have only two sources: factual ignorance as to relevant laws or as to just which properties are present in a situation, or inferential error, such as when conclusions are drawn carelessly from the laws and descriptions of properties.''[35]

However, on this view some very important aspects of particulars are left out. Particulars include such things as salt marshes, planetary systems, dolphins, cities and people, that is, they can occupy a region of space, persist through time, have boundaries, be affected by environment, etc. Every particular exists by virtue of the operation of some set of physical and chemical mechanisms whose description reliably yields the particular. In this manner we build up an account of generalizations about particulars that in turn have great reliability.

The power of these generalizations has led some who think that all genuine scientific knowledge is of universals to suppose that all particulars are of this kind. But Gorovitz and MacIntyre argue that this is clearly false.

> Many particulars—salt marshes, hurricanes, and the higher primates, for example—cannot be understood solely as the sum total of the physical and chemical mechanisms that operate on them. What effects such mechanisms have are affected by the unique history of that contingent specific particular with all its circumstances, contingent, that is, and even accidental, relative to the operation of the mechanisms. One cannot expect therefore in the case of such particulars to be able to move from a theoretical knowledge of the relevant laws to a prediction of the particular's behavior. The history of the law-governed mechanisms and of the particular which is their bearer is, so to speak, an intervening variable which may always to some degree elude us.[36]

In other words, in order to understand some particulars it is not enough to understand their general characteristics, but one must also understand their history.

This means that no one salt marsh is quite like any other salt marsh, nor is any one hurricane like any other hurricane. Perfect knowledge of one particular hurricane is unavailable and this ignorance is not due to ignorance of the initial conditions or of relevant laws, but of the contingencies of the environmental context that can differ from one hurricane to another. In other words, for that kind of particular where the particular's history is crucial the theoretical knowledge of the mechanism of the particular will never be adequate for explanatory or predictive purposes since the conditions of the ideal environment presupposed by the theoretical knowledge will never adequately match the actual conditions (though at times it may be very close).

What is true of hurricanes and salt marshes is also true of animals and people. Of course, it can be objected that the scientist is not interested in those aspects of particulars that do not provide the law-like generalizations of relevance for theoretical science. But that only serves to heighten the difference between such science and practical sciences like meteorology and veterinary medicine. For the latter is not only interested in the similarities that support generalizations, but more importantly what is distinctive about individual hurricanes, cloud formations, or cows. "How such particulars differ from one another in their diversity thus becomes as important as the characteristics they commonly share. Experience of a single entity over time is necessary for an understanding of that entity as a particular in all its distinctiveness, for its individual characteristics will not typically be inferable simply from what is known about the general characteristics of the type of entity of which it is an instance."[37]

Thus the concentration of natural science on knowledge of universals has blinded us to the existence of particulars as proper objects of knowledge. More important for our purposes, however, is that we have been blinded to the role of a type of generalization that is different from the law-like generalizations of the natural sciences. What we must face is that the kind of predictability of those sciences dealing with particulars is more like the predictability of practical or historical inference, rather than that of pure theoretical science.

This has two important implications for activities that deal with explanations and predictions involving particulars. First, it must be seen that a concern for certain values other than those belonging to truth-seeking and problem-solving is internal to practical science. To understand a particular we must understand it from the perspective of its striving for conditions that allow it to flourish. Secondly, it helps us see that error may arise from the present state of scientific ignorance or from negligence, but it may also arise from the necessary fallibility rooted in our knowledge of particulars. For the knowledge of a particular means that we cannot anticipate certain contingencies that are part of the very nature of the particular's existence.

3.1 Implications for Medicine

If MacIntyre and Gorovitz's argument has been correct, it has important implications for the morality of medicine. The first implication is conservative, since their analysis reinforces the view that the physician's concern to have knowledge of the individual patient is essential to medical practice. In other words, it is not just good personal medicine to "know" the patient, it is epistemologically a necessity.

But at the same time it requires a potentially revolutionary view of medical care, since the knowledge of the individual patient is necessarily always potentially inadequate. This means that damaging error may result from conscientious, well-motivated clinical intervention by the best-informed physician. As patients, we are encouraged to think that our physician will not make a mistake, but we must learn to recognize that medicine and the individual physician are necessarily fallible. The physician is committed to the patient's flourishing; but that does not mean the physician may not only fail to cure; he may even damage a patient without violating the canons of the best medicine. (A further implication that would take us too far afield is the status of the distinction between experimental and therapeutic medicine. For if the above is correct, every therapeutic intervention is an experiment in respect to that individual patient.)[38]

This means that while injury may be proof of culpability, it is not necessarily so. We may be hurt from medical therapy where no one is at fault. But what would it mean for us to recognize this? The implications for malpractice are of course immense. But even more important are the implications for the kind of ethos that would support doctor and patient alike as they undergo the healing process. Their mutual knowledge of error—nonculpable error— would seem to require each to have convictions that would sustain the burden of caring that may have tragic results.

The physician's commitment to his patient is not enough to sustain medicine as a moral activity. Nor is it sufficient, as MacIntyre and Gorovitz suggest, for us to take a more humble view of the power of medicine to heal. Rather what is needed is a story that can help us contain the tragic without trying to explain it away or find a "solution" for it. Such a story requires the sustenance of a community with a tradition that knows how to deal with the limits of our existence. But, as we will see in the next section, that is exactly what we do not have.

3.2   Error and Fate in Medicine

Indeed, modern medicine has seemed to embody exactly an opposite story about the nature of human existence. For medicine has been sustained by a story that has as its purpose to eradicate or at least to mitigate as completely as possible the fact of chance from our lives. Chance is fate and fate is death. The goal of autonomy and freedom makes us enemies of chance.

It is important to note, however, that in this respect medicine is in harmony with the major ethical positions of our day. For chance or fate to the modern ethicist represents an irrational surd. We all know that morality must have to do only with those matters that we can do something about. Control, not chance, is the hallmark of the moral man.

However, we should at least remember that for the Greeks it was chance or fate that they took to be central to the moral life. It was the man who knew how to respond to his fate appropriately who was the truly moral man. In the Christian tradition the category of fate also found a place, but it was transformed by the use of the language gift, that is, as grace. Only the man who knows how to accept a gift could be on the road to becoming a good man for he had the moral basis to understand he was not under the power of indifferent fate but rather subject to Providence.

Because we have lost the moral importance of the sense of gift we do not have the skill to deal with tragedy. To lack this skill is only to involve us further in the deceptive story that we can be—or at least should strive to be—free from fate. Thus, as Eric Cassell points out, the most common source of error in medicine is not venality or ignorance.

but in the inherent belief and value structure of medicine equally shared— as must be the case by both physicians and patients. Where the belief exists that fate in its expression as illness can be denied or overcome and where cure is the expectation, there exists a force to act. Medicine is based on a belief in the efficacy of intervention. The focus of the force to intervene is the disease. It is difficult but necessary to point out the difference between disease as entity and disease as symbol. It is clear that the symbolic utility of disease as the carrier of illness is dependent on its concrete utility in individual cases . . . We live in a surgical age in medicine based on a belief in efficacy of the extirpation of disease. It is essential to remember that for the symbol to retain its force both patient and doctor must believe in it. It is from this symbolic meaning of disease and surgery that most error in medicine derives. Patients who have unnecessary hysterectomies are not usually dragged kicking and screaming to the operation room. Both they and their surgeons believe in the importance of the operation. A force exists for its presence. To eliminate that source of necessary surgery it is almost necessary to eliminate surgery. Put another way, the proven efficacy of surgery has as its inevitable accompaniment unnecessary surgery.[39]

Our very urge to control our fate through the office of medicine only makes us more determined by our fate which comes through the office of medicine. What we must do if we are to respond adequately to our fate, a fate that comes through our own will, is to know how simply to recognize the inherent tragedy that is the result of all attempts to care. For example, Cassell points out that at one time it was thought to be the best medicine to keep patients in bed for long periods after surgery. This led to a high incidence of thrombophlebitis and pulmonary emboli. The results of our bad knowledge were tragic in many cases, but it was not anyone's fault.[40]

Moreover, this perspective on tragedy should help us deal with the kind of dilemmas to which MacIntyre alludes in the opening quote. For our difficulty with such matters is that morally we lack the skills to describe what happens in such dilemmas—especially since the dilemmas result from our own power of intervention. Because we lack a sense of the tragic we are tempted to try to justify what we do in such circumstances by using the language of the good—"It is a good thing that we let the child die." But what we must learn to see is that this is to misdescribe the situation by giving in to our need for moral justification. We must simply learn that often in such situations there is no right or wrong thing to do—whatever we do will involve both. Such situations are tragic and we only pervert ourselves and our medical practice if we try to describe them in terms that deny that they are anything else.

What we must learn to do is accept that medicine, like almost all other aspects of our lives, involves trade-offs that are unhappy. There is no way to avoid that. We will take the goods it offers, and they are great goods, but at the same time doctors and patients alike must be willing to accept their losses. And they are hard losses, as they may at times involve life itself. Such losses are tragic, but they can be lived with. They only become destructive when we refuse to recognize them for what they are.

We should accept medicine both for its opportunities and disadvantages, because all good communities must have institutions that gesture that communities care for one another. One of the institutions that we use for that gesture in our society is medicine, but the question is whether we have a sufficient community ethos to sustain and justify the losses that necessarily must accompany our setting apart that role.

4. Medicine as a Tragic Profession

It is time to return to the beginning. I began by suggesting that we could make headway on what we mean by the claim that medicine is a moral art if we attended to MacIntyre's suggestion that medicine is a tragic profession. I have tried to argue that medicine necessarily involves a sense of tragedy, since inherent to its practice is the commitment to sustain life under less happy conditions. Moreover, this very commitment, subject to the boundaries of finitude, necessarily results in errors that often increase our difficulties rather than alleviate them.

Moreover, I suggested that our contemporary social and moral context does little to help us sustain medicine as a tragic profession. As a result, medicine presents an easy target for those like Illich who use the negative results of modern medicine as an argument against its existence. I have tried to suggest that such arguments fail to see that all medicine, including our modern medicine, must necessarily fail, for a success commensurate to our desire is impossible. In this respect I do not mean uncritically to defend modern medicine, but rather to simply point out that morally it is not so different from the folk medicine that Illich seems to prefer.[41]

However, I take no comfort from this conclusion. If I have been right, then I think that we are indeed in a very dangerous time. For if medicine requires a moral community sufficient to sustain it as a tragic profession, then no such community seems to exist. In other words, I am suggesting that no moral community exists to provide medicine with a story sufficient to guide and sustain its activities.[42] As a result, other stories will give it direction that may be dangerous not only to our physical health but more importantly to our moral health.

It would certainly be foolish, as MacIntyre suggests, to try to offer a "solution" to this kind of problem. However, I am equally sure that we cannot make any progress at all as a community until we cease telling ourselves false stories about the nature and power of medicine, and instead attend to how the practice of medicine, like ethics itself, can help us learn to face the tragic nature of our existence. Then medicine would qualify as a truly moral art.

Notes

INTRODUCTION

1. For example see Wes Robbins' criticism of me in his "On the Role of Vision in Morality," and my response, "On Learning to See Red Wheelbarrows: On Vision and Relativism," *Journal of American Academy of Religion*, June, 1977.

2. Bernard Williams, *Morality: An Introduction to Ethics* (New York: Harper Torchbooks, 1973), pp. 1–39.

3. William Frankena, "Reply to Carney and Hauerwas," *Journal of Religious Ethics*, 3 (Spring, 1975), 45–62.

4. Richard Adams, *Watership Down* (New York: Avon Books, 1972) El-ahrairah says to Lord Frith on returning to his warren to discover the rabbits have forgotten the stories of their ancestor's struggle, "I am not angry. But I have learned that with creatures one loves, suffering is not the only thing for which one may pity them. A rabbit who does not know when a gift has made him safe is poorer than a slug, even though he may think otherwise himself," p. 285.

5. H. R. Niebuhr, *The Responsible Self* (New York: Harper & Row, 1963), pp. 59–60.

1: FROM SYSTEM TO STORY

1. For example, James Gustafson ends his recent Marquette Lecture, "The Contributions of Theology to Medical Ethics," by saying "For most persons involved in medical care and practice, the contribution of theology is likely to be of minimal importance, for the moral principles and values needed can be justified without reference to God, and the attitudes that religious beliefs ground can be grounded in other ways. From the standpoint of immediate practicality, the contribution of theology is not great, either in its extent or in its importance" (p. 94). While we have no wish to challenge this as a descriptive statement of what pertains today, we think we can show that even though "moral principles can be justified without reference to God," how they are accounted for still makes a difference for the meaning of the principle and how it works to form institutions and ways of life that may have practical importance. To be sure, Christians may have common moral convictions with non-Christians, but it seems unwise to separate a moral conviction from the story that forms its context of interpretation. Moreover, a stance such as Gustafson's would seem to assume that medicine as it is currently formed is the way it ought to be. In this respect, we at least want to leave open the possibility of a more reformist if not radical stance.

2. We wish to thank Professor MacIntyre for helping us clarify these issues. As will be obvious to anyone acquainted with his work, we are deeply influenced by his argument that the "conflict over how morality is to be defined is itself a moral conflict. Different and rival definitions cannot be defended apart from defending different and rival sets of moral principles." "How To Identify Ethical Principles," unpublished paper prepared for the National Commission for the Protection of Human Subjects of Biomedical and Behavioral Research, p. 8.

3. The search for ethical objectivity, of course, is also a response to the social and political diversity of our day. Thus the search for a "foundation" for ethics involves the attempt to secure rational agreement short of violence. The attraction of the ideal of science for ethicists may be due partly to science appearing to be the last form of universal culture we have left. Of course, this strategy comes to grief on the diversity of activity and disciplines that constitute what we generally call science. For example, see Ernest Becker's reflection on this in his *The Structure of Evil* (New York: Braziller, 1968). The desire for "objectivity" in ethics, moreover, is part of the irrepressible human desire to think that what we have done or had to do is the right thing to do. The quest for certainty, both intellectually and morally, is the need to secure our righteousness in an ambiguous world.

4. We do not mean to claim the actual practice of science involves this sense of objectivity. Indeed we are very sympathetic with Toulmin's analysis of science, not as a tight and coherent logical system, but "as a conceptual aggregate, or 'population', within which there are—at most—localized pockets of logical systematicity." *Human Understanding,* (Princeton: Princeton University Press, 1972), p. 128. It is exactly his stress on necessity of understanding the history of the development of a discipline in order to understand its sense of "rationality" that we feel must be recovered in science as well as, though with different significance, in ethics. As he suggests, "In science as much as in ethics the historical and cultural diversity of our concepts gives rise to intractable problems, only so long as we continue to think of 'rationality' as a character of particular systems of propositions or concepts, rather than in terms of the procedures by which men change from one set of concepts and beliefs to another" (p. 478). Rather, what must be seen is that rationality "is an attribute, not of logical or conceptual systems as such, but of the human activities or enterprises of which particular sets of concepts are the temporary cross-sections" (p. 133).

5. Eric Cassell, "Preliminary Exploration of Thinking in Medicine," *Ethics in Science and Medicine,* 2, 1 (1975), 1–12. MacIntyre and Gorovitz's "Toward a Theory of Medical Error" also obviously bears on this issue. See it in H. T. Englehardt and D. Callahan (eds.), *Science, Ethics and Medicine,* (Hastings-on-Hudson: Hastings Center Publication, 1976).

6. Quoted by B. F. Skinner in *Science and Human Behavior* (New York: Macmillan, 1953), pp. 18–19. Eric Cassell's, "Illness and Disease," *Hastings Center Report,* 6, 2 (April, 1976), 27–37, is extremely interesting in this respect. It is his contention that we as yet have failed to appreciate the obvious fact that doctors do not treat diseases but patients who have diseases.

7. Skinner, p. 19. In the light of Skinner's claim it is interesting to reflect on John Wisdom's observation in *Paradox and Discovery* (New York: Philosophical Library, 1965). "It is, I believe, extremely difficult to breed lions. But there was at one time at the Dublin zoo a keeper by the name of Mr. Flood who bred many lion cubs without losing one. Asked the secret of his success, Mr. Flood replied, 'Understanding lions.' Asked in what consists the understanding of lions, he replied, 'Every lion is different.' It is not to be thought that Mr. Flood, in seeking to understand an individual lion, did not bring to bear his great experience with other lions. Only he remained free to see

each lion for itself'' (p. 138). We are indebted to Professor Ed Erde for the Tolstoy and Wisdom quotes.

8. We are aware that this judgment would need to be qualified if each of these positions were considered in detail. Yet we think that this does characterize a tendency that these positions share. For each position is attempting to establish what Frankena calls the "institution of morality," that is, to show that morality is an institution that stands on its own, separate from other human activities such as politics, religion, etiquette. (We suspect connected with this attempt to establish the independence of ethics is the desire to give ethics a disciplinary character like that of the sciences. For an excellent discussion of ethics as a "quasi-discipline" see Toulmin, *Human Understanding*, pp. 406–411.) The language of obligation tends to become central for these interpretations of the moral life as they trade on our feeling that we ought to do our duty irrespective of how it affects or relates to our other interests and activities. Obligation and rationality are thus interpreted in interdependent terms as it is assumed that an ethics of obligation can provide the standpoint needed to establish the independence of moral discourse from all the relativities of interests, institutions and commitments save one, the interests of being rational. That is, the moral life, at least as it involves only those obligations that we owe one another apart from any special relationships, needs no further grounding apart from our common rationality. It should be obvious that our criticisms of this approach have much in common with such thinkers as Foot, MacIntyre, Toulmin and Hampshire. For a critique of the emphasis on obligation to the exclusion of virtue in contemporary accounts of the moral life see Hauerwas, "Obligation and Virtue Once More," *Journal of Religious Ethics*, 3, 1 (Spring, 1975), 27–44 (and included in this book), and the response and critique by Frankena in the same issue.

9. *Mind*, 80 (1971), 552–571. For similar criticism, see Hauerwas, *Vision and Virtue: Essays in Christian Ethical Reflection* (Notre Dame, Ind.: Fides, 1974).

10. To our mind one of the most disastrous aspects of the standard account of rationality is the resulting divorce of ethical reflection from political theory. It may be objected that the works of Rawls and Nozick are impressive counters to such a claim. However, it is interesting to note that the political theory they generate exists in a high level of abstraction from the actual workings of the modern state. It is only when ethicists turn their attention to C. B. MacPherson's challenge to the liberal democratic assumptions that Rawls and Nozick presuppose that they will address questions that are basic. For liberal political theory and the objectivist's account of moral rationality share the assumption that morally and politically we are strangers to one another. Thus any common life can only be built on our willingness to qualify our self-interest in order to increase our long-term satisfaction. From this perspective the standard account can be viewed as an attempt to secure a basis for rational politics for a society that shares no interests beyond each individual increasing his chance for survival. It is our hunch that historically the disputes and disagreements in ethical theory such as that between Rawls and Hare will appear as scholastic debates within a liberal framework. For the disputants agree on far more than they disagree. For MacPherson's critique of these assumptions see his *Democratic Theory* (Oxford: Clarendon Press, 1973). For a radical critique of liberal democracy both in terms of the liberal understanding of rationality and the self similar to our own, see Roberto Unger's, *Knowledge and Politics* (New York: Free Press, 1975).

11. For a critique of this assumption see Michael Walzer, "Political Action: The Problem of Dirty Hand," *Philosophy and Public Affairs*, 2, 2 (Winter, 1973), 160–180. He is responding to Hare's "Rules of War and Moral Reasoning," *Philosophy and Public Affairs*, 1, 2 (Winter, 1972), 161–181. Hare argued that though one might

wrongly think he was faced with a moral dilemma this could not be the case if a course of action suggested itself that was moral. See also John Ladd's very useful discussion of this issue in his "Are Science and Ethics Compatible?" in Engelhardt and Callahan (eds.), *Science, Ethics and Medicine*. This is also the issue that lies behind the theory of double effect in Roman Catholic moral theology though it is seldom explicitly discussed in these terms. For example, see Richard McCormick's, *Ambiguity in Moral Choice* (Marquette Theology Lectures: Marquette University, 1973). See Hauerwas, "Natural Law, Tragedy, and Theological Ethics," included in this volume, for a different perspective.

For a fascinating study of the problem of moral evil in terms of the economic category of scarcity, see Vivian Walsh, *Scarcity and Evil* (Englewood Cliffs: Prentice-Hall, 1961). Ms. Walsh argues that we are often mistaken in trying to ascribe responsibility for actions that are the result of scarcity even when the scarcity is not the result of the "external" limits but in the person doing the action. What we often must do is the lesser good because of our own limits, but we must learn to know it is a lesser good without implying that we are morally blameworthy. Even though we are sympathetic with Ms. Walsh's analysis, we think the concept of character provides a way to suggest what is an inappropriate "scarcity" for anyone to lack in their character given the form of their engagements. Albert Speer lacked political sense that became morally blameworthy because of his political involvement, but that does not mean morally there is no way to indicate that his character should have provided him with the skills to know what kind of politics he was involved with. In classical terms the concept of character gives the means to assess in what ways we are blameworthy or praiseworthy for what we have omitted as for what we have "done."

12. For a discussion of these issues see Hauerwas, "The Demands and Limits of Care: Ethical Reflections on the Moral Dilemma of Neonatal Intensive Care," included in this volume.

13. It is not just Prichard that argues in this way but, as Henry Veatch suggests, Kant is the primary inspiration behind those that would make interest, desires and beliefs, in principle, unjustifiable. This, of course, relates to the matter discussed in note 4, as Kant wanted to provide a basis for morality not dependent on any theological or anthropological assumption—except that of man's rational capacity. That is why Kant's principle of universalizability, which has so often been misinterpreted, applies only to men as rational beings and not to just all human beings. As Veatch points out in this latter case, "the maxim of one's action would be based on a regard simply for certain desires and likings characteristic of human nature—albeit desires that all human beings happen to share in. But any mere desire of inclination or liking or sentiment of approbation, even if it be shared by the entire human race, would still not be universalizable in the relevant sense, simply because it was something characteristic of and peculiar to human kind, and hence not truly universal." "Justification of Moral Principles," *Review of Metaphysics*, 29, 2 (December, 1975), 225.

14. For example, witness this exchange between Lucy and Linus as Lucy walks by while Linus is preparing a snowball for launching.

LUCY: Life is full of Choices.
        You may choose, if you so wish to throw that snowball at me.
        You may also choose, if you so wish not to throw that snowball at me.
        Now, if you choose to throw that snowball at me I will pound you right into the ground.
        If you choose not to throw that snowball at me, your head will be spared.

LINUS: *(Throwing the snowball to the ground)* Life is full of choices, but you never get any.

15. For a more extended analysis of the concept of character, see Hauerwas, *Character and the Christian Life: A Study in Theological Ethics* (San Antonio: Trinity University Press, 1975). For a similar critique of the Kantian inspired moral philosophy, see Bernard Williams, "Person, Character, and Morality," in Amelie Rorty (ed.), *The Identities of Persons* (Berkeley: University of California Press, 1976), pp. 197–215.

16. Julius Kovesi, *Moral Notions* (New York: Humanities Press, 1967), and Hauerwas, *Vision and Virtue,* pp. 11–29. For a detailed account of how the meaning of a word depends on its history, see Raymond Williams, *Keywords* (New York: Oxford, 1976).

17. For example, R. S. Downie and Elizabeth Telfer attempt to argue that "the ordinary rules and judgments of social morality presuppose respect for persons as their ultimate ground . . . [and] that the area of private or self-referring morality also presupposes respect for persons as its ultimate ground." *Respect for Persons* (New York: Schocken, 1970), p. 9. They interpret respect for persons in a Kantian fashion of respecting the claim another rational capacity—that is, capable of self-determining and rule-governing behavior—can demand. It never seems to occur to them that the "ordinary rules of social morality" or "self-referring morality" may not need an "ultimate ground." Moreover, they have a good deal of trouble explaining why we owe respect to children or "idiots" on such grounds. They simply assert that there "are sufficient resemblances between them and persons" to justify extending respect to them (p. 35). For a different perspective on this issue, see Hauerwas, "The Retarded and the Criteria for the Human," included in this volume. It is Downie and Telfer's contention that "respect for persons" is the basis of such Christian notions as agape. It is certainly true that much of what a "respect for persons" ethic represents has been assumed by Christian morality, but we think that it is misleading to assume that the story that informs the latter can be translated into the former. One of the places to see this is how each construes the relationship between obligation and supererogation. The Christian ethic of charity necessarily makes obligatory what a follower of "respect for persons," can see only as supererogation. For an analysis of agape in terms of equal regard, see Gene Outka, *Agape: An Ethical Analysis* (New Haven: Yale University Press, 1972).

18. For an account of the moral life that makes "fittingness" central, see H. R. Niebuhr, *The Responsible Self* (New York: Harper and Row, 1963).

19. It would take us too far afield to explore this point further, but surely it is Kant that stands behind this understanding of the self. It is impossible to document this, but it is at least worthwhile calling attention to two passages from *Religion Within the Limits of Reason Alone,* translated by Theodore Green (New York: Harper, 1960). "In the search for the rational origins of evil action, every such action must be regarded as though the individual had fallen into it directly from a state of innocence. For whatever his previous deportment may have been, whatever natural causes may have been influencing him, and whatever these causes were to be found within or outside him, his action is yet free and determined by none of these causes; hence it can and must always be judged as an original use of his will. . . . Hence we cannot inquire into the temporal origins of this deed, but solely into its rational origin, if we are thereby to determine and, whereby possible, to elucidate the propensity, if it exists, i.e., the general subjective ground of the adoption of transgression into our maxim" (p. 36). In case it is objected that Kant is only dealing with moral evil, consider "To reconcile the concept

of freedom with the idea of God as a *necessary* Being raises no difficulty at all: for freedom consists not in the contingency of the act, i.e., not in indeterminism, but rather in absolute spontaneity. Such spontaneity is endangered only by predeterminism, where the determining ground of the act is in *antecedent time,* with the result that, the act being now no longer in my power but in the hands of nature, I am irresistibly determined; but since in God no temporal sequence is thinkable, this difficulty vanishes'' (p. 45). It is, of course, the possibility of the moral law that Kant thinks gives men the possibility to be like God—timeless. It is not a far distance from Kant to the existentialist in this respect. Of course it is true that the Kantian outlook, as Williams suggests, makes less of an abstraction of the individual than utilitarianism. But the question arises ''of whether the honourable instincts of Kantianism to defend the individuality of individuals against the agglomerative indifference of Utilitarianism can in fact be effective granted the impoverished and abstract character of persons as moral agents which the Kantian view seems to impose.... It is a real question, whether the conception of the individual provided by the Kantian theories is in fact enough for others who, while equally rejecting Utilitarianism, want to allow more room than Kantianism can allow for the importance of individual character and personal relations in moral experience.'' Bernard Williams, ''Persons, Character, and Morality,'' in A. Rorty (ed.) *The Identities of Persons,* pp. 200–201.

20. For this point and much else that is involved in this paper, see Iris Murdoch, *The Sovereignty of the Good Over Other Concepts* (Cambridge: Cambridge University Press, 1967).

21. We have not based our criticism of the standard account on the debates between those who share its presuppositions. It is, of course, true that as yet no single theory of the standard account has proved to be persuasive to those who share its presuppositions. We still find Kant the single most satisfying statement of the program implied by the standard account.

22. Ernest Becker, however, argues that Comte has been misunderstood as his purpose was not to free science from morality but to call attention to what kind of moral activity science involved. Thus Becker suggests, ''Comte's Positivism, in sum, solved the problem of science and morals by using science to support a man-based morality. With all the force at his command he showed that life is a moral problem, and science only a tool whose unity would serve the larger unity of life. Like de Maistre and de Bonald, and like Carlyle in England, he looked approvingly on the Middle Ages. But he did not pine nostalgically for their institutions; he saw the Middle Ages as possessing what man needed most, and has since lost: a critical, unitary world view by which to judge right and wrong, good and bad, by which to subordinate personal desire to social interest. But instead of basing this knowledge on theological fiat, man could now settle it firmly on science. In this way, the Enlightenment could achieve what the Middle Ages almost possessed; but it could do this on a much sounder footing than could ever have been possible during the earlier time, namely, it could achieve the subordination of politics to morality on a scientific rather than on a theological basis. Social order and social harmony would be a call of the new day, and human progress could then be progress in social feeling, community, and love—all of it based on the superordinate science of man in society, serving man, elevating humanity.'' *The Structure of Evil,* p. 50.

In this respect, consider Simone Weil's observation that ''The criticism of religion is always, as Marx said, the condition for all progress; but what Marx and the Marxists have not clearly seen is that, in our day, everything that is most retrograde in the spirit of religion has taken refuge, above all, in science itself. A science like ours, essentially closed to the layman, and therefore to scientists themselves, because each is layman outside his narrow specialism, is the proper theology of an ever increasingly bureaucratic society.''

23. Cf. G. E. M. Anscombe, ''Thought and Action in Aristotle,'' in R. Bambrough (ed.), *New Essays on Plato and Aristotle* (New York: 1965), pp. 151-152. See also Hauerwas, *Character and the Christian Life,* Chapter II.

24. For an account of the way analogous terms can be used once they are effectively linked to a paradigm instance, cf. Burrell, *Analogy and Philosophical Language* (New Haven and London: Yale University Press, 1973).

25. It may of course happen that one cannot sustain a particular relationship and ''fails.'' Again, the way he deals with that becomes a story. Stories often seem better the more they overturn conventional assessments and challenge settled attitudes.

26. Peter Brown shows how this choice represented an existential decision as well. The *Platonici* formed an identifiable group of noble humanists, and as such offered a viable alternative to Christianity. While they were not formed into a church, their common aspirations could well be imagined to constitute a community of like-minded persons. See, *Augustine of Hippo* (Berkeley: University of California Press, 1967).

27. This is the point of Peter Winch's oft-cited analysis: ''Understanding a Primitive Society,'' reprinted in Bryan R. Wilson (ed.), *Rationality* (Oxford, 1970).

28. For further elaboration of this, see Iris Murdoch, *The Sovereignty of the Good Over Other Concepts.*

29. Cf. James Cameron's efforts to offer perspective to current writing on the ''sexual revolution,'' in *New York Review of Books,* 23 (May 13, 1976), 19-28.

30. MacIntyre's argument in ''Towards a Theory of Medical Error,'' that medicine must necessarily deal with explanations of individuals only makes this claim more poignant. For the attempt to claim that the only errors in medicine were those characteristic of a science of universals was necessary if medicine was to make good its claim to be the means to free mankind of the limits of disease. To recognize that medical explanation and prediction is subject to the same limits as explanation and prediction of individuals will require a radical reorientation of the story that morally supports and directs medical care.

31. Becker, *The Structure of Evil,* p. 18. ''The central problem posed by the Newtonian revolution was not long in making itself felt. This was the momentous new problem; it is still ours today—I mean of course the problem of a new theodicy. If the new nature was so regular and beautiful, then why was there evil in the human world? Man needs a new theodicy, but this time he could not put the burden on God. Man had to settle for a new limited explanation, an anthropodicy which would cover only those evils that allow for human remedy.'' Science naturally presented itself as the ''remedy.''

32. It is tempting to try to make, as many have, the ethic of ''respect for persons'' sufficient as a moral basis for medical care. (Cf. Paul Ramsey's *The Patient as Person.*) But if, as we suggest, medicine is necessarily involved in tragic choices, a more substantive story than that is needed to sustain and give direction to medical care. Without such a story we will be tempted to make technology serve as a substitute as it allows us to delay further decisions of life and death that we must make in one or another arena. For a critique of the way ''person'' is being used as a regulative moral notion in medical ethics, see Hauerwas, ''Must a Patient Be a 'Person' To Be a Patient, or My Uncle Charlie is Not Much of a Person But He Is Still my Uncle Charlie,'' included in this volume.

33. For an analysis of the concept of self-deception, see Burrell and Hauerwas, ''Self-Deception and Autobiography: Theological and Ethical Reflections on Speer's *Inside the Third Reich,*'' included in this volume.

34. Jules Henry's analysis of the phenomenon of "sham" is perhaps the most graphic depiction of this. He says,

Children in our culture cannot avoid sham, for adults cannot escape depression, hostility and so on. Since sham consists in one person's withholding information, while implying that the other person should act as if he had it all; since sham consists also in giving false information while expecting the other person to act as if the information were true; since sham consists in deriving advantage from withholding or giving information—and since, on the whole, our culture is sham-wise, it might seem that the main problem for the mental health of children is to familiarize them with the edges of sham. Yet, if we were to do that, they would be "shot" for Albee is right. Our main problem, then, is to tell them the world lies but they should act as if it told the truth. But this, too, is impossible, for if one acted as if all sham were truth he might not be shot, but he certainly would lose all his money and marry the wrong person though he would have lots of friends. What then is the main problem; or rather, what does mankind do? People do not like children who lack innocence, for they hold the mirror up to adults. If children could not be deceived, they would threaten adults beyond toleration, they would never be orderly in elementary school and they clearly could not be taught the rot-gut dished out to them as truth. Personally I do not know what to do; and I anticipate a geometric increase in madness, for sham is at the basis of schizophrenia and murder itself (*On Sham, Vulnerability, and Other Forms of Self-Destruction* [New York: Vintage Books, 1973], pp. 123–124).

See also his *Pathways to Madness* (New York: Vintage Books, 1971), pp. 99–187.

35. For a fuller development of the issues in this last section see Hauerwas, "Natural Law, Tragedy, and Theological Ethics," included in this volume. Moreover, for a perspective similar to this see Ernest Becker, *The Denial of Death* (New York: Free Press, 1975). In a broad sense Becker suggests man's situation is tragic because, "Man has a symbolic identity that brings him sharply out of nature. He is a symbolic self, a creature with a name, a life history. He is a creator with a mind that soars to speculate about atoms and infinity, who can place himself imaginatively at a point in space and contemplate bemusedly his own planet . . . yet at the same time man is a worm and food for worms. This is the paradox: He is out of nature and hopeless in it; he is dual, up in the stars and yet housed in a heart-pumping, breath-grasping body that once belonged to a fish. Man literally is split in two: he has awareness of his own splendid uniqueness in that he sticks out of nature with a towering majesty, and yet he goes back into the ground a few feet in order blindly to rot and disappear forever. It is a terrifying dilemma to be in and to have to live with" (p. 26).

36. In his *Revisioning Psychology* (New York: Harper & Row, 1975), chapter 1, James Hillman questions whether psychic integration has not been conceived in too "monotheistic" a manner. His discussion is flawed by failing to see how an analogical "reference to one" offers a feasible way of mediating between an ideal which is too confining and a *laissez faire* program which jettisons ideals altogether.

2: OBLIGATION AND VIRTUE ONCE MORE

1. William K. Frankena, "Prichard and the Ethics of Virtue," *Monist*, 54 (January, 1970), 17. Fortunately, this essay and some of the others cited below (" 'Ought' and 'Is' Once More," "Obligation and Motivation in Recent Moral Philosophy," and

"On Saying the Ethical Thing"), appeared in the excellent new collection of Frankena's occasional essays *Perspectives on Morality: Essays by William K. Frankena,* edited by Kenneth E. Goodpaster (Notre Dame, Ind.: University of Notre Dame Press, 1976).

2. The line of argument I develop in this paper obviously owes much to such philosophers as Foot, Anscombe, Hampshire, MacIntyre, Murdoch and Williams.

3. Frankena, "Prichard . . . ," *Monist,* p. 4.

4. Frankena, " 'Ought' and 'Is' Once More," *Man and World,* 2 (November, 1969), 515. Here he is quoting Dewey.

5. B. O. A. Williams, "A Critique of Utilitarianism," in J. J. C. Smart and Bernard Williams, *Utilitarianism: For and Against* (Cambridge: Cambridge University Press, 1973), pp. 108–118.

6. Frederick S. Carney, "The Virtue-Obligation Controversy," *Journal of Religious Ethics,* 1 (1973), 5–19.

7. Stanley Hauerwas, *Vision and Virtue: Essays in Christian Ethical Reflection* (Notre Dame, Ind.: Fides, 1974). Also *Character and the Christian Life: A Study in Theological Ethics* (San Antonio: Trinity University Press, 1975).

8. See especially "Prichard . . . ," *Monist,* pp. 9–10. Also "The Ethics of Love Conceived as an Ethics of Virtue," *Journal of Religious Ethics,* 1 (Fall, 1973), 21–36.

9. Frankena, "The Ethics of . . . of Virtue," *Journal of Religious Ethics,* p. 24.

10. Hauerwas, *Character and the Christian Life,* chapter III.

11. "Prichard . . . ," *Monist,* p. 6.

12. Ibid.

13. "The Ethics of . . . of Virtue," *Journal of Religious Ethics,* p. 32.

14. For an extended analysis of Aristotle on this point, see Hauerwas, *Character and the Christian Life,* chapter II.

15. "Prichard . . . ," *Monist,* p. 7.

16. Frankena, "Under What Net?" *Philosophy,* 49 (1973), 320. In the language of Rawls, Frankena is concerned to give basic obligations the force of what Rawls calls natural duties—i.e., those duties which we have irrespective of any voluntary or institutional context. John Rawls, *A Theory of Justice* (Cambridge: Harvard University Press, 1971), pp. 114–117.

17. "The Ethics of . . . of Virtue," *Journal of Religious Ethics,* pp. 26, 32.

18. "Prichard . . . ," *Monist,* p. 10.

19. Ibid., p. 13.

20. Frankena, "Obligation and Ability," in Max Black (ed.), *Philosophical Analysis* (Ithaca, N.Y.: Cornell University Press, 1950), p. 159.

21. For a fuller discussion of this issue see Hauerwas, *Character and the Christian Life,* chapter III.

22. Thomas Aquinas, *Summa Theologica,* Fathers of the English Dominican Province (transl.), (University of Chicago: Great Books Publishing Co., 1952), II, 20, 2.

23. "Prichard . . . ," p. 11.

24. "The Ethics of . . . of Virtue," pp. 25, 31.

25. Ibid., p. 24.

26. Frankena, "Prichard . . . ," p. 11.

27. Frankena, "The Ethics of . . . of Virtue," p. 30.

28. "Educating for the Good Life," in H. E. Kiefer and M. K. Munitz (eds.), *Perspectives in Education, Religion, and the Arts* (Albany: State University of New York Press, 1970), p. 30.

29. Frankena, "The Ethics of . . . of Virtue," p. 32.

30. Ibid., p. 33.

31. Frankena, "Prichard . . . ," p. 15.

32. Ibid., p. 14.

33. Julius Kovesi, *Moral Notions* (New York: Humanities Press, 1967), p. 54.

34. Richard Norman, *Reasons for Action* (New York: Barnes and Noble, 1971), pp. 63–64.

35. Frankena, "Obligation and Motivation in Recent Moral Philosophy," in A. I. Melden (ed.), *Essays in Moral Philosophy* (Seattle: University of Washington Press, 1958), pp. 73–74.

36. Ibid., p. 44; also Frankena, "Ought and Is Once More," *Man and World,* p. 516.

37. Frankena, *Ethics,* 2nd ed. (Englewood Cliffs, N.J.: Prentice-Hall, Inc., 1973), p. 70.

38. Frankena, "Toward a Philosophy of Moral Education," *Harvard Educational Review,* 28 (1958), 308.

39. Frankena, "On Saying the Ethical Thing," *Proceedings and Addresses of the American Philosophical Association,* 39 (1966), 32.

40. Ibid., p. 33.

41. "Ought and Is Once More," *Man and World,* p. 528.

42. Stuart Hampshire, "Morality and Pessimism," *The New York Review of Books,* January 25, 1973, p. 29.

43. Ibid., p. 19.

44. Ibid., p. 29.

45. Ibid., p. 40.

46. Ibid.

47. Ibid.

48. Frankena, "Recent Conceptions of Morality," in H. N. Castaneda and G. Nakhnikian (eds.), *Morality and the Language of Conduct,* (Detroit: Wayne State University Press, 1963), p. 9; also Frankena, "The Concept of Morality," *University of Colorado Studies in Philosophy,* No. 3 (1967), p. 158. [Reprinted in G. Wallace and A. Walker (eds.), *The Definition of Morality.* This is an earlier version of "The Concept of Morality," *Journal of Philosophy,* 63 (November 10, 1966), 688–696. Reprinted in K. Pahel and M. Schiller (eds.), *Readings in Contemporary Ethical Theory.*]

49. Frankena, "On Saying the Ethical Thing," *Proceedings and Addresses . . . ,* pp. 23–33.

50. Frankena, "The Concept of Morality," *Journal of Philosophy,* 63 (November 10, 1966), 691, 695.

51. Frankena, "Recent Conceptions of Morality," *Morality and the Language of Conduct,* p. 19.

52. *Man and World,* 2 (November, 1969), 515–533.

53. Ibid., p. 525.

54. Ibid., p. 529; also Frankena, "Obligation and Motivation . . . , *Essays in Moral Philosophy,* p. 50.

55. "Ought and Is Once More," *Man and World,* p. 529.

56. Ibid., p. 530; also Frankena, "On Saying the Ethical Thing," *Proceedings and Addresses . . . ,* p. 39.

57. Frankena, "Ought and Is Once More," *Man and World,* p. 530.

58. Frankena, "On Saying the Ethical Thing," p. 38.

59. Hauerwas, *Vision and Virtue;* also Iris Murdoch, *The Sovereignty of Good* (New York: Schocken Press, 1971).

60. David Burrell and Stanley Hauerwas, "Self-deception and Autobiography: Theological and Ethical Reflections on Speer's *Inside the Third Reich,*" included in this volume.

61. Frankena, "Recent Conceptions of Morality," *Morality and the Language of Conduct,* pp. 1–2.

62. Frankena, "Is Morality Logically Dependent on Religion?" in Gene Outka and John P. Reeder (eds.), *Religion and Morality* (Garden City, N.Y.: Anchor Books, 1973), pp. 195, 314–316.

63. I would like to thank Rev. Ed Malloy, Rev. David Burrell, Ken Goodpaster, Richard Bondi and Jim Childress for reading and criticizing earlier drafts of this paper. I owe a particular debt to Professor David Solomon for sharpening and suggesting how my argument might be developed.

3: NATURAL LAW, TRAGEDY AND THEOLOGICAL ETHICS

1. For an excellent analysis of this debate and its relation to natural law, see Rev. Edward Malloy's *Contemporary Catholic Appropriations of H. R. Niebuhr's Ethics of Responsibility* (Ph.D. Thesis: Vanderbilt University, 1975). Fr. Malloy points out that the critique of natural law involves claims that natural law (1) is not scriptural; (2) involves static and unhistorical understanding of man's existence; (3) is used to bolster positions and conclusions arrived at on other grounds; (4) tends toward a physicalist interpretation of human activity, and (5) proposes an inflated number of negative absolutes. Most of these criticisms have been countered by pointing out that the classical understanding of natural law has little relation to how natural law was understood and applied in the textbooks. Through a recovery of Aquinas there is a new emphasis on the rational character of natural law and the contingent character of most of the principles of natural law. See for example Michael Crowe, "Natural Law Theory Today," in Dan Berjene and James McGlynn (eds.), *The Future Ethics and Moral Theology* (Chicago: Argus Communication Co., 1968), pp. 78–105.

2. For example, we are told that natural law must be reinterpreted to satisfy the "contemporary thrust of morality [that] is in the direction of an ethics of responsibility in which the dynamic, historical, concrete, empirical, personal elements are more and more coming to the fore." Thomas Wassmer, *Christian Ethics for Today* (Milwaukee: Bruce, 1969), p. 77. Why this "contemporary thrust" is assumed normative or how it can be satisfied is not explained. Behind such statements is a valid pastoral concern, but unfortunately the pastoral issue is thought to determine the theoretical question of the status and objectivity of moral norms and judgments. It is interesting to notice that just at the time many Catholics are rejecting natural law many Protestant theologians are finding it a renewed source of wisdom. For example, see Douglas Sturm's arguments that natural law does not necessarily deny the significance of history, in "Naturalism, Historicism, and Christian Ethics: Toward a Christian Doctrine of Natural Law," in Martin Marty and Dean Peerman (eds.), *New Theology,* No. 2 (New York: Macmillan, 1965), pp. 77–96. Moreover, Frederick Carney argues most persuasively that natural law can be defended against most of the philosophical and theological objections brought against it; see his "Outline of a Natural Law Procedure for

Christian Ethics," *Journal of Religion,* 47, 1 (January, 1967), 26–38. David Little has
dealt with many of the same objections in his very important article, "Calvin and the
Prospects for a Christian Theory of Natural Law," *Norm and Context in Christian
Ethics,* pp. 175–197. Finally, Paul Ramsey must be mentioned as one of the first
Protestant moralists who reopened the question of natural law for recent work in
theological ethics. In particular, see his *Nine Modern Moralists* (Englewood Cliffs,
N.J.: Prentice-Hall, 1962).

3. In this respect arguments about the significance of natural law often take the form
of ideological commitments. The failure to appreciate the importance of natural law is
alleged to be the cause of the moral relativism, if not immorality, of our times, e.g.,
the loss of natural law leads straight to mercy killing, abortion, and Auschwitz. Even
as sophisticated a thinker as Germain Grisez at times moves unaccountably from
metaethical arguments to ethical or political conclusions in this way. Grisez, however,
has clearly developed one of the most consistent as well as persuasive theories of
natural law. See in particular his "First Principle of Practical Reason: A Commentary
on Summa Theologiae, 1–2, Question 94, article 2," *Natural Law Forum,* 10 (1965),
168–201. Defenders of natural law have an unfortunate tendency to criticize the
weakest possible statement of their adversaries' position. For example, natural law
thinking often involves some form of consequentialist reasoning, especially as it is
bounded by a teleological ethical framework, yet defenders of natural law dismiss
utilitarianism for being consequentialist. There is an important issue between advocates of natural law and utilitarianism, but it is not where the defenders of natural law
usually locate it. Rather, the issue involves the utilitarian assumption that the moral life
is fundamentally a matter of balancing one value against others. In contrast, natural
law rightly involves the claim that some values cannot be so balanced, as they are the
necessary presuppositions for any balancing to take place—in other words, no basic
value can be abrogated in order to achieve higher values without perverting the nature
of the moral life. This is not, however, the same issue as whether there are unexcep-
tionable or "absolute" moral rules. On this latter issue see the essays in Paul Ramsey
and Gene Outka (eds.), *Norm and Context in Christian Ethics* (New York: Scribners,
1968); and Donald Evans, "Paul Ramsey on Exceptionless Moral Rules," *American
Journal of Jurisprudence,* 16 (1972), 184–214.

4. For this sense of convictions and how they can be true and false see James
McClendon and James Smith, *Understanding Religious Convictions* (Notre Dame: U.
of Notre Dame Press, 1975). For them "A 'conviction' is persistent belief such that if
X (a person or a community) has a conviction, it will not easily be relinquished and it
cannot be relinquished without making X a significantly different person than before."
In particular see their Chapter IV where they analyze "conviction sets."

5. This type of theological ethics tends to be associated with what Troeltsch identified as the "Church type." This type of Christianity is world-affirming as Christians
are encouraged to participate fully in the affairs and institutions of secular society. In
such a context natural law functions ideologically to justify the assumption that Christians have a responsibility to fulfill the demands of the state and institutions associated
with it. It is no accident, therefore, that "natural law" as a doctrine flourished during
the Constantinian era of the church. The content of natural law becomes identified with
the "humanism" of a particular historical period. As a result the church has sometimes
assumed it has a stake in the continuation and perpetuation of historically relative
institutions. Even though Christians often do and will share much with their non-
Christian neighbor, it is my opinion that when this is turned into a matter of principle in
the name of natural law, it comes close to perverting the nature of the Christian life.

My own ecclesiology is closer to what Troeltsch called the "sect type" which means I assume that Christians will always be in fundamental tension with secular society. Therefore, natural law is not a commitment to finding what all men can agree about, but rather an attempt to show how the commitments incumbent on Christians may enliven the form of the moral life of any man. At the very least this kind of issue should remind us that natural law cannot be separated from ecclesiological and sociological assumptions.

6. For this sense of story see my *Vision and Virtue: Essays in Christian Ethical Reflection* (Notre Dame: Fides, 1974), pp. 68–89. Briefly put, a story is the narrative structure necessary to display the conviction set of our lives.

7. Richard McCormick, "Human Significance and Christian Significance," *Norm and Context in Christian Ethics*, pp. 233–261.

8. George Regan, *New Trends in Moral Theology* (New York: Newman Press, 1971), pp. 130–131. Fuchs, for example, says "natural law is an abstraction from the total reality which is Christian man." *Natural Law* (New York: Sheed and Ward, 1965), xi. Of course, involved with these systematic points is the further claim of the magisterial office of the church authority to determine the natural law. I will not deal with this issue at all; for a good analysis, see J. P. Mackey, "Teaching Authority in Faith and Morals," in J. P. Mackey (ed.), *Morals, Law and Authority*, (Dayton: Pflaum, 1969), pp. 91–114.

9. McCormick, p. 241.

10. Bruno Schüller, "Can Moral Theology Ignore Natural Law?" *Theological Digest*, 15 (1967), 96. The influence on Schüller and the positions above of Rahner's anthropology and its implications for how the relation of nature-grace is understood is obvious.

11. The status of such claims is extremely unclear to me. I fail to understand what difference such "ontological" concerns make for how one understands moral argument, rules or how the moral virtues are formed and ordered.

12. Paul Ramsey, *Nine Modern Moralists*, p. 4.

13. Ibid., p. 5. The systematic concern of this essay is perhaps most often raised in the Protestant context as the question of the relation of justice and love, agape and eros. One must be careful in this respect, however, as these may be quite different questions. For an excellent analysis of how the debate about "law" usually appears in terms of the Protestant concern for the relation between law and gospel, see Edward Long, "Soteriological Implications of Norm and Context," *Norm and Context in Christian Ethics*, pp. 265–295.

14. N. H. G. Robinson, *The Groundwork of Christian Ethics* (Grand Rapids: Eerdmans Publishing Company, 1971), p. 86.

15. Ibid., p. 122. In another context Robinson articulates well the kind of tension always characteristic of Christian ethics.

Men are moral beings apart from Church and Scripture, and when Christian thought takes the form of Christian ethics it does not lead men into an entirely new country where a quite different language has to be learned, it does not land on the moon but enters a field already occupied. The Christian is certainly *in some sense* a new creature, but that clearly means, not another species altogether, but a creature, a man transformed or renewed, whose transformation and renewal cannot be articulated apart from some understanding of his existence as a creature independently of that renewal. No more then can the ethical side of that transformation be understood apart from some comprehension of the human condition which is the subject of renewal. In other words, Christian ethics cannot get under way in any adequate and fundamental fashion unless it comes to terms with, and related itself to, natural man's understanding of his own moral existence, his own existence as a man. (p. 16. Italics mine.)

Statements such as this make it clear why phrases like "in some sense" should be prohibited for use by theologians.

16. Though I would want to argue that if the law is rightly understood, how argument and rules function in law is similar to morality. For example, see Frederick Carney, "The Role of Rules in Law and Morality," *Southwestern Law Journal* (1969), pp. 438–453. Also see Gideon Gottlieb, *The Logic of Choice* (New York: Macmillan, 1968), for an extraordinarily perspicacious account of the relation between rules and rationality using law as a paradigm.

17. See, for example, my "Obligation and Virtue Once More," included in this volume.

18. See my *Character and the Christian Life: A Study in Theological Ethics* (San Antonio: University of Trinity Press, 1975).

19. Indeed, it seems that the failure to understand this was the primary difficulty with Roman Catholic moral theology. By attempting to find a standpoint to secure the objectivity of moral judgments devoid of all characteristics of agents, moral theologians necessarily tended to give a minimalist interpretation of the moral life. The religious life thus appeared as a further "topping" to the moral life; religion was something "added to" but not fundamentally affecting one's moral existence. In such a context moral theology became too rationalistic as it assumed or attempted to secure a special epistemological status for certain values prior to an agent's moral formation and commitments. I will suggest below why the principle of double effect becomes the crucial question for such an ethics. More research is needed for it seems such an ethic is at odds with major voices in Roman Catholic tradition. For example, in his "The Ethical Theory of St. Thomas," *The Journal of Religion*, 50, 2 (April 1970), 169–185, L. Thiry points out the importance of virtue and character for Aquinas' thought: "Virtue being a stable disposition of character that makes the performance of good actions easy and joyful, the central question in ethics is for him not 'what shall I do?' but rather, 'what kind of a person shall I be?' . . . the emphasis in Thomistic ethics is not on the enumeration of permitted and forbidden actions but in the problem of how to become truly human" pp. 179–181.

Connected with the minimalist type of moral theology is the issue discussed in footnote 5. The church type encourages the attempt to do moral theology from the perspective of "every man." Thus, the theologian does not expose his theological convictions until there is no other recourse. If the argument of this essay is right, however, this is a fundamental mistake. While it is certainly true that the Christian and the man of goodwill may share much in common, the area of commonality methodologically does not warrant the Christian ethicist to write his ethics as though the convictions of Christians are an afterthought to the moral life. Christian ethics is written for Christians, not for all men. This is not just a statement of who one's audience is, but a fundamental methodological point. Aquinas' insistence that charity must be the form of the virtues seems to me to support this point. Unfortunately, many have taken Aquinas' distinction between the natural and theological virtues more seriously than Aquinas' own analysis allows for. Indeed, Aquinas insists as strongly as Augustine that "natural virtues" are but "a false likeness to virtue." *Summa*

Theologica, translated by the Fathers of the English Dominican Province (Chicago: Encyclopaedia Britannica, 1952), II–II, 23, 7.

20. Peter Geach, "The Moral Law and the Law of God," *God and the Soul* (New York: Schocken Books, 1969), pp. 117–129. The problem is, many seem to assume that if this is admitted, then religious convictions can add nothing to "morality." This is, however, to give a far too restrictive interpretation of "morality." Much of the debate surrounding the religion–morality problem has been due to the failure to appreciate this point. However, for an excellent collection of essays on this problem, see Gene Outka and John Reeder (eds.), *Religion and Morality* (Garden City: Anchor Books, 1973).

21. For example, see Aquinas, *Treatise on Law* (Chicago: Gateway Edition, 1967).

22. James A. Weisheipl, one of Aquinas' recent biographers, discusses this problem on page 260 of his *Friar Thomas D'Aquino: His Life, Thought and Work* (New York: Doubleday, 1974), as follows: "Unfortunately, many modern commentators have wrenched Thomas's teaching on natural law out of context and have distorted it; similarly, certain aspects of his teaching on grace have been distorted. Frequently they fail to see that Thomas's approach is derived from St. Augustine's *De spiritu et littera,* and *De natura et gratia.* The discussion of law in general and of the natural law in particular does not constitute Thomas's full teaching on the foundations of natural law. In I–II, these are only preliminary questions for his principal interest, which is the Old Law and the New Law of the covenant which God made with his people."

23. Bernard Williams, *Morality: An Introduction to Ethics* (New York: Harper Torchbooks, 1973), p. 56.

24. Ibid., p. 54. For an example of what happens when such dissociation does not happen, see Burrell and Hauerwas, "Self-Deception and Autobiography: Theological and Ethical Reflections on Speer's *Inside the Third Reich,*" included in this volume.

25. Robert Jay Lifton, *Boundaries* (New York: Vintage Books, 1969), p. 44.

26. Williams, p. 57. In the past a sense of honor served to manifest a sense that men thought of themselves as having a self apart from their roles. An indication of the character of our society is that cynicism is made to do the work of honor. For an account of how the loss of honor has implications for the university see my "Truth and Honor: The University and the Church in a Democratic Age," in *The Proceedings of the James Montgomery Hester Seminar* (Winston-Salem: Wake Forest University, 1976), pp. 33–53.

27. "Rationality" is, of course, not just a "role" but also a capacity, indeed a capacity that we cannot be without. However, appeals to "rationality" or the mark of man are not just descriptive appeals to what we are, but rather normative claims about what we should be (a role). As will be evident below, my emphasis on agency functions in much the same way—i.e., agency is a capacity that also serves as a role description of what men should be. Natural law claims about the good of man being rooted in his "nature" are best interpreted in this sense—namely, that certain of our capacities make intelligible certain kinds of roles. However, the logic of these claims has often been confused insofar as certain roles have been said to be necessarily or unavoidably embodied in our rational capacity.

28. Aristotle, *Nicomachean Ethics,* translated by Martin Ostwald (Indianapolis: Bobbs-Merrill, 1962), pp. 1144a24–1144a37. Williams rightly argues that Aristotle did not provide "any account of how the intellectual activities, the highest expression (in his view) of man's nature, are to be brought into relation to the citizenly activities which are regulated by the virtues of character." *Morality,* p. 60. Williams also

criticizes Aristotle's emphasis on rationality as the mark of man because (1) rationality can be used for evil as well as good and (2) rationality emphasizes self-control at the expense of all else. These criticisms, are, however, clearly matters of perversion that are not necessarily implied by Aristotle's position. See, for example, Ralph McInerny's response in his "Naturalism and Thomistic Ethics" (unpublished paper).

Though it is not often noticed, Aquinas was as insistent as Aristotle that practical reason must be directed by the virtues if it was to function properly. In order "for a man to do a good deed, it is requisite not only that his reason be well disposed by means of a habit of intellectual virtue, but also that his appetite be well disposed by means of a habit of moral virtue," *Summa Theologica*, I–II, 52, 2.

29. I owe this point to Dr. David Solomon.

30. This may be one of the few contexts where the is-ought issue becomes relevant for the analysis of natural law.

31. For an effective criticism of this model of rationality, especially as it takes a utilitarian form, see Stuart Hampshire, "Morality and Pessimism," *New York Review of Books*, 11 (January 25, 1973), 26–34. Because proponents of natural law often are critical of utilitarianism, it is overlooked that some natural law positions, especially as they stress norms derived from the need of survival, share many of the utilitarian assumptions about the nature and functions of reason within our life scheme.

32. The attempt to ground justice in the character of "rationality" itself perhaps has received its strongest formulation in Rawls, *A Theory of Justice* (Cambridge: Harvard, 1971). Even though I am impressed by Rawls' attempt to ground a nonutilitarian view of justice in our "rational" capacity, I am not convinced a substantive account of justice can be so derived. For such a concept of justice continues to treat individuals as units of preference rather than beings who can and should form their lives in accordance with the best that they know. Indeed Rawls even takes this a step further and asks us to view ourselves as strangers; that to be moral we must separate ourselves from our projects. In such a scheme alienation from self becomes the fundamental moral virtue on which all other moral concerns are based. Thus, for Rawls, like the utilitarians, the agent's moral task is to view each of his projects from an observer's point of view. Not only does this prevent a viable theory of the self, but as Milton Fisk observes, it makes it difficult to account for community. "Mutual disinterestedness and the awareness that one has fellow feeling toward unspecified fellows cannot be combined to form a coherent conception of human nature. . . . Community is possible only when, from the start, there are individual powers that have been recognized and 'organized' as social powers." "History and Reason in Rawls Moral Theory," in Norman Daniels (ed.), *Reading Rawls* (New York: Basic Books, 1975), p. 65.

33. Charles Fried, "Reason and Action," *Natural Law Forum*, 11 (1966), 13–35; see note 32.

34. Charles DeKoninick, "General Standards and Particular Situations in Relation to Natural Law," *Situationism and the New Morality* (New York: Appleton-Century-Crofts, 1970), pp. 217–218. This is, of course, but a restatement of Aquinas' insistence that a "requisite for prudence, which is right reason about things to be done, that man be well disposed with regard to the ends, and this depends on the rectitude of his appetite. Therefore, for prudence there is need of a moral virtue, which rectifies the appetite." *Summa Theologica*, I–II, 57, 4. See also 59, 5 and 65, 1 and 2. This point makes clear, as I argued above, why it is so misleading to read the "Treatise on Law" as if it is Aquinas' definitive position on "natural law." Rather, his view of "natural law" is much more determined by his analysis of the virtues than of the "external principles" of law. I suspect that "natural law" becomes a particularly misleading

phrase in the theological context exactly because it seems to signal the attempt to secure the objectivity of external and coercive norms that all men share irrespective of their theological convictions. To interpret Aquinas as attempting to defend such a view of natural law is to fail to do justice to his primary concern with how men do what they ought to do in order that in doing what they ought to do they do it in a manner that they become good men—i.e., men of character. Vernon Bourke argues in a similar fashion that "the theory of right reason seems to me to take precedence over the theory of natural law" in Aquinas' ethics. "Is Thomas Aquinas a Natural Law Ethicist?" *The Monist*, 58, 1 (January, 1974), 510–66. I would only add that "right reason" could be as misleading as "natural law" if it is separated from Aquinas' analysis of human activity and virtue.

35. For an analysis of how destructive even the most humane attempts to settle on a criterion for the human can be, see my "The Retarded and the Criterion for the Human," included in this volume.

36. McCabe, *What Is Ethics All About?* (Washington: Corpus Press, 1969), p. 57.

37. Dorothy Emmet, *Rules, Roles, and Relations* (New York: Macmillan, 1966), p. 179.

38. Charles Fried, "Natural Law and the Concept of Justice," *Ethics*, 74 (July, 1964), 244. Fried's emphasis on action is a return to Aristotle's and Aquinas' central emphasis.

39. For a further analysis and defense of this distinction, see my *Character and the Christian Life*, Chapters II and III. I have attempted to use the language of "reason" in this essay, but as should be clear from my other works the concept of "agency" is more basic. Rationality is for me, as I think it was also for Aquinas, but another way of talking about agency.

40. Fried, "Natural Law and the Concept of Justice," p. 244.

41. "The idea of rationality is that of the ability, given certain present and particular data, to unite or relate them with other data in certain appropriate ways," Jonathan Bennett, *Rationality* (New York: Humanities Press, 1964), p. 85.

42. "The happy life is regarded as a life in conformity with virtue," Aristotle, *Nicomachean Ethics*, 1177a1–2.

43. Ralph McInerny, "Ultimate End in Aristotle." Unpublished paper, p. 17.

44. There are important questions whether *eudaimonia*, even interpreted in the most compelling manner, is a sufficient summary image for the life of Christians. I suspect the Christian way of ordering the virtues to meet the demands of charity requires much greater risk of suffering than a "happiness" ethic can ever admit.

45. Lon Fuller, *The Morality of Law* (New Haven: Yale University Press, 1964), pp. 185–186. As Herbert McCabe says, "Man does not just *add* speech on to such things as eating and sexual behavior; the fact that these latter occur in a linguistic context makes a difference to what they are," *What Ethics Is All About*, p. 68.

46. For this interpretation of Calvin, see David Little, "Calvin and the Prospects for a Christian Theory of Natural Law," *Norm and Context in Christian Ethics*, pp. 175–197; and Frederick Carney, "Associational Thought in Early Calvinism," in D. B. Robertson (ed.), *Voluntary Associations* (Richmond: John Knox Press, 1966), pp. 39–53.

47. Put in more theological language, our lives are only sustained within covenantal frameworks. As Jews and Christians we do not believe that we exist if we have status independent of the covenant God has made with us and our fellows. Rather, our existence is fundamentally a gift—i.e., we are creatures. The social nature of our existence is, therefore, but a form of our creatureness.

48. Knud Lögstrup, *The Ethical Demand* (Philadelphia: Fortress, 1971), pp. 8–9.
See James Childress' insightful commentary on this passage in his "Nonviolent Resistance: Trust and Risk Taking," *Journal of Religious Ethics,* Fall 1973, pp. 87–94. In
this connection, perhaps one of the most important questions for any society is how it
identifies and treats the stranger. As Richard Titmuss suggests, "the ways in which
society organizes and structures its social institutions—and particularly its health and
welfare systems—can encourage or discourage the altruistic in man; such systems can
foster integration or alienation; they can allow the 'theme of gift'—of generosity
towards strangers—to spread among, and between social groups and generations."
The Gift Relationship (New York: Vintage Books, 1971), p. 225. The justice of a
society is, therefore, not to be gauged primarily by how equitably it distributes its
material goods or values, but rather how open it is to supporting the strangers in its
midst, especially as they appear as the weak.
   49. I am obviously using the language of "promise" analogously since the kinds of
promises I am concerned with are primarily implicit. I will not attempt to work this
analogy out in detail, but rather am content to point out that much of our life involves
implicit promises that have become so much a part of us we no longer notice them.
   Moreover, as Julian Hartt points out, "Promises are not necessarily moral," since
we may promise many things that are immoral to carry out. For example, "I promise
to knock your block off" is not a morally good promise to keep in most circumstances.
However, the argument I am trying to develop does not deny that individual promises
may be immoral, but rather that promising as an institution is crucial for the trust
morally necessary to sustain human existence. As Hartt goes on to say, "We ought not
to doubt that there are many ways by which promises can be deficiently rational and
fall short of the ethical. But it would be wrongheaded to infer that the promise as such
is incompatible with the ethical as such. Surely there is moral weight to keeping one's
word, other things being equal. A moral weight and not just a prudential one. Trust is
the foundation of much else in the moral life. Indeed trustworthiness can be achieved
quite independent of promise giving. I may say, 'I will do the best I can to see justice
done,' but that is not a promise; I am simply telling you what my intentions are and
indicating that I resolve to stand by them. A person who so comports himself is
trustworthy. Here it is the performance along the lines of the posted intentions that
creates certain expectations. You may well be disappointed if I let you down but you
do not have an enforcable claim against me." *The Restless Quest* (Philadelphia:
Pilgrim Press, 1975), pp. 154–155.
   50. Lisa Perkins, "Natural Law in Contemporary Analytic Philosophy," *The
American Journal of Jurisprudence,* 17 (1972), 118. Ms. Perkins rightly criticizes
Searle and Veatch for treating the self-involving character of language as if it were an
optional characteristic of our existence. Bennett, in a similar way, argues "that language would become impossible in the absence of a general inclination toward truthfulness." *Rationality,* p. 70.
   The view, I have defended elsewhere, that ethics is a form of therapy whose task is to
help a community keep its grammar pure gets its full sense in this context. See my
"The Ethicist as Theologian," *Christian Century,* 92, 15 (April 23, 1975) pp. 408–
412.
   51. Fried, "Natural Law and the Concept of Justice," p. 246. I remain unconvinced by Fried's further argument that Rawls' two criteria of justice can be derived
from this analysis of man's sociality and ability to act. Thus, Fried argues, "By the
norm of human nature a person in his dealings with others may not deny either his own
or any other person's capacity for free and rational action. To do so is always to act

irrationally—that is, a failure to make a true judgment of reality and ground of one's acts—and therefore to act contrary to one's nature" (248). For a quite different attempt to ground "other regardingness" in the character of practical reason, see Thomas Nagel's *The Possibility of Altruism* (Oxford: Clarendon Press, 1970). I would prefer to say that the understanding of "rationality" I have sketched makes it intelligible to say that one ought to view his neighbor's interest as equal to his own, or perhaps even more important than his own, but we cannot claim he is irrational for not doing so. In other words, I do not think rational explanations can be given for holding rational beliefs. Indeed, it is a mistake to assume rational beliefs need or can have any further ground than their own rationality. I simply do not find convincing those Kantian-inspired interpretations of morality that try to ground morality in "rationality" abstracted from the dispositions, convictions, and cares that give direction to our lives morally. However, for a fuller statement of Fried's position see his *An Anatomy of Values* (Cambridge: Harvard University Press, 1970).

I am, moreover, aware that the claim that man's nature is social is open to challenge on anthropological grounds. Works such as Colin Turnbull's *The Mountain People* (New York: Simon and Schuster, 1972) certainly make one hesitate to claim that men are naturally social beings. However, I think one of the striking things about Turnbull's study is that when people become divorced from one another they become divorced from themselves, and lose interest in everything beyond barest survival. Moreover, my argument does not entail that people will be always trustworthy. I know that the conditions of trust are less than ideal in many of our societies; that, for example, it is unsafe to walk at night in many of our cities. The necessity of man's sociality and trustworthiness serves rather to remind us that this is not as it should be, indeed, that such unfaithfulness is conceivable only because we are bound together by a deeper humanity.

52. Yet as E. A. Goerner has argued, this point has mistakenly been used to argue that democracy is necessarily the most appropriate form of political life: "Aristocracy and Natural Right," *The American Journal of Jurisprudence*, 17 (1972), 1–13. Moral equality cannot be automatically translated into political equality, especially when the latter takes the form of the individualistic assumptions of liberal democracy. As should be clear, the strong claims of man's sociality implied in my view place me in tension with the individualistic assumptions of some forms of democratic liberalism.

53. See, for example, my discussion of the rule against lying in *Vision and Virtue*, pp. 87–89.

54. Albert Jonsen, "Natural Law Anew" (unpublished talk), p. 9. See also his *Christian, Decisions, and Actions* (Milwaukee: Bruce, 1970), pp. 149–150; and his and Edward MacKinnon's, "A Reinterpretation of Natural Law Ethics," *The American Catholic Philosophical Association Proceedings*, 1970, pp. 161–170. Also see James Gustafson, "The Moral Conditions Necessary for Human Community," *Christian Ethics and the Community* (Philadelphia: Pilgrim Press, 1971), pp. 153–163, for an approach very similar to the one taken here. Gustafson uses faith, hope, and love as the prerequisites for community. To start with these virtues, however, seems to be somewhat circular since these virtues are singled out because of a prior understanding of community that is not a "requisite." However, I would not deny that my own account may involve the same kind of circularity even though I have tried to provide a more extensive account than Gustafson of how faithfulness and honesty are required by our nature as social and language-using creatures. However, like Gustafson, I do not think that faithfulness and honesty are necessarily sufficient for sustaining our life. I have chosen to emphasize them simply because they seem to have an immediacy that is

hard to question. For a more extended discussion of Gustafson's position, see my review essay of "Christian Ethics and the Community" in *Reflection*, 69, 3 (March, 1972), 9–14.

55. This seems to provide the basis for a "natural law" interpretation of law, but so understood it is unclear how this differs from any attempt to understand the interaction of law and custom. See, for example, Burton Leiser, *Custom, Law and Morality* (New York: Anchor Books, 1969).

56. Augustine, *The City of God,* translated by Marcus Dodds (New York: Modern Library, 1950), pp. 19, 25, See also, "On the Morals of the Catholic Church," in Philip Schaff (ed.), *Nicene and Post-Nicene Fathers of the Christian Church*, IV, (New York: Scribner's Sons, 1901), p. 6. For a more extended analysis of how virtues can be vices without Augustine's theistic assumptions, see Alasdair MacIntyre's "How Virtues Become Vices: Values, Medicine and Social Context," in Tristram Engelhardt and Stuart Spicker (eds.), *Evaluation and Explanation in the Biomedical Sciences* (Utrecht, Holland: Reydal, 1975); Vol. I, Series in Philosophy and Medicine, pp. 97–111.

57. Augustine, "On the Morals of the Catholic Church," 15, 25. It is just such a quote that reveals the significance of character for the Christian ethical reflection. For character is the "role" that gives all our other "roles" their characteristic form and direction. Or perhaps better "love" is not just a virtue that informs the other virtues, but it is the conviction that God loves me and the policy that is built into and responds to that conviction. I am indebted to Professor James McClendon for this formulation of the matter.

58. Fried, "Reason and Action," pp. 32–33. In another context, Fried argues that physicians have a special obligation to care for the individual patient though such a commitment may not work out in the best interest of the greatest number. But then he suggests, "We must reduce the suffering of men, but not so much because suffering is bad, as because it is human beings who are suffering. Consequently, it is more important that we retain respect for our own and each other's humanity as we relieve suffering, than that suffering be relieved. After all suffering like death will always be with us." *Medical Experimentation: Personal Integrity and Social Policy* (New York: American Elsevier Pub., 1974), p. 140. This is a succinct summary of one of the major points of this essay. I am contending, however, that what we require is a story that helps us continue to act morally in such a world without the suffering that remains stilling our moral activity or turning it to unwarranted idealism that would rid the world of all suffering or an equally disastrous cynicism that has lost the patience to act in a finite world.

59. However, see Ramsey, *Nine Modern Moralists*, pp. 245–256.

60. Fried, "Natural Law and the Concept of Justice," p. 249.

61. At this point there is a certain similarity between my position and Germain Grisez's. The difference lies, I think, in the fact that I assume that the goods of human life may conflict, whereas Grisez seems to think that it cannot possibly happen morally that in order to have one good one must turn against another.

62. Moral tragedy is distinguished from tragedy by the fact that the lesser evil must be willed as part of the moral act. Most tragedies or calamities do not raise moral questions so directly.

63. The commitment of the pacifist is but a particularly intense form of the necessary shape of the moral life. For pacifism rightly construed is not the attempt to protect life irrespective of all other commitments but rather the willingness to die rather than have to use immoral means to protect life. See, for example, John Howard Yoder, "What Would You Do If," *Journal of Religious Ethics*, 2 (Fall, 1974), 81–106.

64. Richard McCormick, *Ambiguity in Moral Choice* (Pere Marquette Theology Lecture: Marquette University, 1973) is the best treatment of this distinction. However, McCormick's position has been brilliantly criticized by Paul Ramsey in a yet unpublished essay. While I remain unconvinced that direct-indirect is finally viable, I am sure that a very limited version of it may be important in order to maintain that human life should never be directly attacked. What bothers me about such formulations is the tendency to make this into a policy that excuses the use of force prior to the action.

65. Theologically the primary problem with utilitarianism is its refusal to face the tragic character of human existence. As such it is a powerful and tempting form of the Pelagian heresy that always tries to convince us that moral goodness can only be sustained in a world where good effects result from acting morally.

66. I wish to thank those who have read an earlier draft of this paper and given me invaluable criticisms. The paper would have been better if I had been able to follow more of their criticisms than I have. They are: Richard Bondi, David Burrell, James Gustafson, Jim Besnahan, Fred Carney, Charles Reynolds, Jim Childress, David Harned, Robert Rodes, Albert Jonsen, Jock Reeder, Edward Malloy, James McClendon, Ed Goerner, and Peri Arnold.

4: STORY AND THEOLOGY

1. "A 'conviction' is a persistent belief such that if x (a person or community) has a conviction, it will not easily be relinquished and it cannot be relinquished without making x a significantly different person than before." James McClendon and James Smith, *Understanding Religious Convictions* (Notre Dame: University of Notre Dame Press, 1975), p. 7.

2. James McClendon, *Biography as Theology* (Nashville: Abingdon Press, 1974), p. 188.

3. Sallie TeSelle, "The Experience of Coming to Belief," *Theology Today*, 32, 2 (July, 1975), 159–160.

4. Hans Frei, *The Eclipse of Biblical Narrative* (New Haven: Yale University Press, 1974), p. 16. The paradigm case of "realistic narrative" is of course the eighteenth-century novel.

5. Doctorow suggests in an interview that "there's no more fiction or non-fiction now, there's only narrative." *Newsweek*, July 14, 1975, p. 76.

6. L. O. Mink, "The Divergence of History and Sociology in Recent Philosophy of History," *Logic, Methodology and Philosophy of Science*, IV (Holland: North-Holland Publishers, 1973), 725–742.

7. As McClendon and Smith suggest, "the justification or rejection of convictions must often consist in the justification or rejection of sets of convictions, of conviction sets, which will stand or fall in interdependence and not one by one . . . The glue which binds convictions into a single set is their mutual relation to the life of the person or (normally) the life of the community in which he shares. The unity of conviction sets is the rough but vital unity of shared life." *Understanding Religious Convictions*, p. 104.

8. "The Ethicist as Theologian," *Christian Century* 92, 15 (April 23, 1975), 408–412.

9. Bernard Williams, *Morality: An Introduction to Ethics* (New York: Harper Torchbooks, 1972), p. 34.

10. George Stroup, "A Bibliographical Critique," *Theology Today*, 32, 2 (July, 1975), 134.

11. The issue of point of view simply raises too many issues to try to develop here. Obviously the truth of a story can depend on from whose perspective it is told. The issue of different perspectives is thus one way to investigate how truth claims about stories can be tested.

12. John Zuck has provided an excellent critique of Frei on this point in his essay "Tales of Wonder: Biblical Narrative, Myth, and Fairy-Stories," *Journal of the American Academy of Religion*, 2 (June, 1976), 299–308.

13. Harold Toliver, *Animate Illusions: Explorations of Narrative Structure* (Lincoln: University of Nebraska Press, 1974), p. 302.

14. By using narrative as the primary mark of story I do not mean to overlook the differences between various kinds of narrative. For attempts to classify narrative see Robert Scholes and Robert Kellogg, *The Nature of Narrative* (London: Oxford University Press, 1966) and Harold Toliver, *Animate Illusions*. Moreover, how indebted the novel is to narrative is a matter of dispute; see, for example, Ted Estess, "The Inerrable Contraption: Reflections on the Metaphor of Story," *Journal of the American Academy of Religion*, 42 (September, 1974), 415–434 and Dale Cannon's excellent response, "Ruminations on the Claim of Inerrability," *Journal of the American Academy of Religion*, 43 (September 4, 1975) 560–585.

15. Elizabeth Anscombe, *Intention* (Oxford: Basil Blackwell, 1958) pp. 9–11.

16. Hayden White, "The Structure of Historical Narrative," *Clio*, 1, 3 (June, 1972), 15.

17. L. O. Mink, "History and Fiction as Modes of Comprehension," *New Literary History*, 1, 3 (1970), 545.

18. The difference between history and fiction is not that one is "literally" true and the other imaginative, but rather that the latter follows a script while the former does not. As Toliver suggests, "The fact is that no historical event follows a preordained and intended script entirely. It is always open to some contingencies and changes of plan that even in the wisest retrospect cannot be accounted for, and there are always uncontrollable perspectives on the event" (*Animate Illusions*, p. 99). But of course that cannot be true of fiction where the world created, even if drawn as an uncontrolled world, is controlled. Interestingly, however, a historian when writing of history must work like the novelist in exercising control over the particular narrative. The difference between them is that the historian's narrative is open to question, i.e., some "events" are left out, in the way the novelist is not. Novelists, however, often testify to how they cannot control their characters—indeed, one of the marks of great literature seems to be the artist's ability to display the contingent character of his tale.

19. Mink, "History and Fiction as Modes of Comprehension," p. 555.

20. Frei, *Eclipse of Biblical Narrative*, pp. 13–14.

21. Scholes and Kellogg, *The Nature of Narrative*, p. 239.

22. Frei, *Eclipse of Biblical Narrative*, p. 13.

23. Steven Crites, "Myth, Story, History," in Tony Stoneburner (ed.), *Parable, Myth, and Language* (Cambridge: Church Society for College Work, 1968), p. 68.

24. TeSelle, "The Experience of Coming to Believe," p. 160.

25. David Burrell, *Analogy and Philosophical Language* (New Haven: Yale University Press, 1973).

26. There is an important lesson in this for theology that I cannot develop here. Briefly, however, it means that theology has lost its way when it attempts to provide a theory of the meaningfulness of religious convictions. The task of theology is primarily

finding the means to remind us what we are or should be doing when we profess adherence to the claim that God has acted graciously through Israel and Christ.

27. Hannah Arendt, *The Human Condition* (New York: Doubleday Anchor, 1958), p. 181.

28. Ibid., p. 286.

29. This, of course, raises great difficulty for if God is an agent who must be known like other agents—that is, through his story—it must also be a story told from his point of view. But we know no such story and must learn of God through others' stories of their relationship with him. Perhaps this is the grammatical context for the claim that some people are his "chosen ones."

30. See, for example, Bob Krieg, *The Theologian as Narrator: Karl Barth on the Perfections of God* (Ph.D. Dissertation, University of Notre Dame, 1976).

31. I am using "go on" here in a normative sense as what the story must do is provide us with the skills to handle the basic ontological invariable of our lives, e.g., fate, anxiety, tragedy, hope and so on.

32. Burrell and Hauerwas, "Self-Deception and Autobiography: Theological and Ethical Reflections on Speer's *Inside the Third Reich*," included in this volume.

33. McClendon and Smith, *Understanding Religious Convictions,* p. 15.

34. Mink, "History and Fiction as Modes of Comprehension," pp. 557–558.

35. McClendon, *Biography as Theology,* pp. 37–38.

36. This has the form of a moral argument for God, not in the sense that if you are to be good you must believe, but in the sense that seeing how things should go in the world implicates the conviction that the world is bounded and supported by a particular kind of God.

5: SELF–DECEPTION AND AUTOBIOGRAPHY

1. David Harned, *Faith and Virtue* (Philadelphia: Pilgrim Press, 1973), pp. 29–30. See also Stanley Hauerwas, *Vision and Virtue: Essays in Christian Ethical Reflection* (Notre Dame, Ind.: Fides Press, 1974).

2. Bernard J. F. Lonergan anticipated this systematic shift in his *Insight* (1957). For an interpretation of Lonergan in this connection, see Burrell, "Method and Sensibility: Novak's Debt to Lonergan," *Journal of American Academy of Religion,* 40 (1972), 349–367.

3. Herbert Fingarette, *Self-Deception* (New York: Humanities Press, 1969), pp. 38–39.

4. Ibid., p. 42.

5. Ibid., p. 47.

6. Henry, *Pathways to Madness* (New York: Vintage Press, 1973).

7. Ibid., p. xviii.

8. Stanley Hauerwas, *Character and the Christian Life: A Study in Theological Ethics* (San Antonio: University of Trinity Press, 1974).

9. Fingarette, p. 140.

10. Albert Speer, *Inside the Third Reich* (New York: Avon Books, 1970) p. 379. Hereafter, all references to this work in the text will be designated simply "Speer" with the appropriate page numbers.

11. For a good analysis of the way truth functions in autobiography, see Pascal, *Design and Truth in Autobiography* (Cambridge: Harvard University Press, 1960), pp.

61–83. He argues that "too scrupulous adherence to the factual truth may injure an autobiography." For the "truth remembered is the only truth that matters—A person's life illusion ought to be as sacred as his skin."

12. H. R. Trevor-Roper, *The Last Days of Hitler* (New York: The Macmillan Co., 1947), p. 75.

13. Hannah Arendt, in *Eichmann in Jerusalem: A Report on the Banality of Evil* (New York: Viking, 1963), p. 253, says, "The trouble with Eichmann was precisely that so many were like him, and that many were neither perverted nor sadistic, that they were, and still are, terribly and terrifyingly normal. From the viewpoint of our legal institutions and of our moral standards of judgment, this normality was much more terrifying than all the atrocities put together, for it implied—as had been said at Nuremberg over and over again by the defendants and their counsel—that this new type of criminal, who is in actual fact *hostis generis humani*, commits his crimes under circumstances that make it well-nigh impossible for him to know or to feel that he is doing wrong."

14. Stuart Hampshire, in *Freedom of the Mind* (Princeton: Princeton University Press, 1971), p. 246, says, "If sincerity is interpreted as undividedness of mind, and if to be sincere in regretting, or to be sincere in one's whole mind, then 'watching oneself live' may be, not an obstacle, but rather a necessary condition of sincerity." Interpreted in this sense, Speer did not have a story from which he could "watch himself live" that was sufficient for the kind of engagement he had begun.

15. In spite of his work against Hitler in these matters, and even with his somewhat halfhearted attempts to kill Hitler, the personal attraction and loyalty Speer felt for Hitler lasted right until the end. For example, see his account of his decision to fly to Berlin for one last meeting with Hitler (p. 606). Speer and Hitler's mutual enthusiasm for architecture formed a bond between them not broken to the end.

16. In response to his daughter's letter asking how an intelligent man like her father could go along with Hitler, Speer says,

let me begin my answer by a confession which is most difficult to make: in my case there is no excuse. The fault is mine, and expiation there must be. . . . Sometimes in the life of a people collective suggestion shows its effect. Man is full of bad instincts which he tries to suppress. But if the barriers once give way, then something dreadful is unleashed. Some few individuals escape the common folly, but when it is all over, and one regains awareness, the world takes its head in its hands and asks: 'How did I come to do it?' Then for me personally there was one factor making for the exclusion of all criticism, if I had wished to express any. You must realize that at the age of thirty-two, in my capacity as architect, I had the most splendid assignments of which I could dream. Hitler said to your mother one day that her husband could design buildings the like of which had not been seen for two thousand years. One would have had to be morally very stoical to reject the prospect. But I was not at all like that. As I have already told you, I did not believe in any God, and that would have been the only possible counterbalance. There was one enormous fault, one which I shared with others. It had become a habit to do one's job without occupying oneself with what the neighbors were doing. By that I wish to say that I did not think it had anything to do with me when somebody else said that all the Jews ought to be wiped out. Clearly I said nothing of this kind, neither did I think like that. I never showed any Anti-Semitism myself, and stayed calm. The fact that I helped many Jews is no excuse. On the contrary, it aggravates the moral fault. More than once I have put myself the question what I would have done if I had felt myself responsible for what Hitler did in other spheres of activity. Unfortunately, if I am to stay sincere, the answer would be negative. My position as an architect and the magnificent projects on which I was engaged became indispensable to me. I swallowed all the rest, never giving it a thought (William Hamsher, *Albert Speer: Victim of Nuremberg* [London: Leslie Frewin, 1970], pp. 65–66).

17. Trevor-Roper, pp. 240–241.

18. Carl Jung, *Civilization in Transition: The Collected Work of C. G. Jung*, Vol. X (1964), 179–193.

19. Hauerwas, *Character and the Christian Life*, see note 8.

20. "Every significant narrative contains images many and various, of course, but among them there are never many that can serve as master images enabling us to grasp concretely and practically what the story means. A master image provides a distillation of a story; among several options, the best is the one that enshrines the most possibilities for articulation of the entire narrative.... Obviously enough, if master images are not themselves qualified and enriched by all the other metaphors in the story, they are not master images at all. The more numerous are the images of the self as moral agent that a narrative provides, the more numerous will be the possibilities for individual life, because we do not intend what we cannot see and imagine ourselves accomplishing. Even so, there still must be a master image that expresses the unity within the variety and that condenses the sprawl and prosody of the narrative into a concrete and powerful metaphor which is able to acquaint the self with the core of whatever the story means." Harned, p. 160.

21. Bernard Lonergan, *Method in Theology* (New York: Herder and Herder, 1972).

22. David Burrell, "Reading *The Confessions* of Augustine: An Exercise in Theological Understanding," *The Journal of Religion*, 50 (October, 1970), 331.

23. Malcolm later found the story that he learned from the Black Muslims also led to illusion because of its inability to countenance men and women of other colors as potential brothers and sisters. His involvement in normative Islam represented another development of his story in his quest for truth.

24. This story allows them even to confess to God sins that they cannot fully understand. Thus one confession reads, "O God, our heavenly Father, I confess unto thee that I have grievously sinned against thee in many ways; not only by outward transgressions, but also by secret thoughts and desires which I cannot fully understand, but which are all known to thee. I do earnestly repent, and am heartily sorry for these my offences, and I beseech thee of thy great goodness to have mercy upon me, for the sake of thy dear Son, Jesus Christ Our Lord, to forgive my sin and graciously to help my infirmities."

25. "Man loves himself inordinately. Since his determinate existence does not deserve the devotion lavished upon it, it is obviously necessary to practice some deception in order to justify such excessive devotion. While such deception is constantly directed against competing wills, seeking to secure their acceptance and validation of the self's too generous opinion of itself, its primary purpose is to deceive, not others, but the self. The self must at any rate deceive itself first. Its deception of others is partly an effort to convince itself against itself. The fact that this necessity exists is an important indication of the vestige of truth which abides with the self in all its confusion and which it must placate before it can act. The dishonesty of man is thus an interesting refutation of the doctrine of man's total depravity." Reinhold Niebuhr, *The Nature and Destiny of Man*, I (New York, Charles Scribner's Sons, 1949), p. 203.

6: MEMORY, COMMUNITY AND THE REASONS FOR LIVING

1. For example, see R. B. Brandt, "The Morality and Rationality of Suicide," in Seymour Perlin (ed.), *A Handbook for the Study of Suicide* (New York: Oxford Press, 1975), pp. 61–75.

2. See, for example, Marvin Kohl, "Voluntary Beneficent Euthanasia" in the book edited by him, *Beneficient Euthanasia* (Buffalo: Prometheus Books, 1975), pp. 130–144. Kohl argues that euthanasia is a positive moral duty insofar as we have an obligation to be kind. That seems a bit odd, as it is not clear why we have an obligation to be kind, kindness usually being associated with those aspects of the moral life which are commendable but not obligatory.

3. On "hard cases" see Sissela Bok, "Euthanasia and the Care of the Dying" pp. 1–25 in John A. Behnke and Sissela Bok (eds.), *The Dilemmas of Euthanasia* (New York: Anchor Books, 1975).

4. For this sense of "background beliefs", see Phillipa Foot, "Moral Beliefs," in Judith Thompson and Gerald Dworkin (eds.), *Ethics* (New York: Harper & Row, 1968), pp. 239–260. We use the language of "story" rather than belief because of its richer connotations. It is not just the "beliefs" we hold about life that form our attitudes toward suicide, but our attitudes are skills that result from the stories that form our lives; that is, beliefs are not self-involving in the same manner as stories.

5. Jack Douglas, *The Social Meanings of Suicide* (Princeton: Princeton University Press, 1967). See especially the appendix, "Formal Definitions of Suicide," where Douglas demonstrates the fundamental dimensions of meaning in definitions of suicide. For a more psychological approach to suicide, see Edwin Shneidman (ed.), *On the Nature of Suicide* (San Francisco: Jossey Bass, 1973). We are aware that the reasons or motives for suicide can be as various as the individuals who commit suicide. The question, however, is how each of us should learn to train our intentions in accordance with the moral commitments involved in the notion of suicide. In other words, the notion, suicide, involves what kind of intentionality we should have about life. The fact that people who commit suicide often have a wide range of reasons does not defeat the meaningfulness of suicide as a moral notion, but rather is a reminder how important it is that we know how to use the notion at all.

6. Arthur Dyke has coined the word "benemortasia" to mean "the ethical framework that one adopts in order to interpret what it is to experience a good death, or at least what would be the most morally responsible way to behave in the face of death, either one's own or that of others." "Beneficient Euthanasia and Benemortasia: Alternative Views of Mercy" in Kohl (ed.), *Beneficient Euthanasia,* pp. 117–129.

7. It is particularly at this point we suggest, that we cannot evade tragedy and suffering. See the argument in section 3.2.

8. It should be clear that nothing we have said or will say indicates whether attempted suicide should or should not be against the law. We have no "in principle" objection to laws against suicide as it may be one of the ways a society gestures its concern for all its members as a society of trust. Of course, some societies may have become such societies of strangers it makes no sense to have such laws. The legal situation with regard to euthanasia is more complicated. See section 3 for a discussion of the relevant problems.

9. Thus the taking of life within the Japanese tradition is not necessarily suicide until we know more about the kind of story that informs their actions.

10. This view of ethics owes much to the work of Alasdair MacIntyre. In particular see his *A Short History of Ethics* (New York: Macmillan, 1966) and *Against the*

Self-Image of the Age (New York: Schocken Books, 1971). In several essays not yet published MacIntyre has developed this position, arguing persuasively that we are inheritors of "fragments" of past moral stories in a manner that makes it impossible to develop any one coherent account of morality. MacIntyre argues that those attempts to provide a formal definition of morality that can in some manner assure the objectivity of moral judgments are, in fact, opting for one moral fragment against others. MacIntyre suggests, therefore, that in order to know the sense of such notions as suicide, murder or stealing, or such virtues as justice, courage or humility, you must know the narrative context in which they are displayed. For example, see his "How Virtues Became Vices: Values, Medicine, and Social Context," in H. T. Engelhardt and S. Spicker (eds.), *Evaluation and Explanation in the Biomedical Sciences* (Utrecht, Holland: Reydal, 1975), pp. 97–111.

11. The work of Adolf Jensen, Mircea Eliade and Claude Lévi-Strauss provides ample evidence of the close relationship between memory and community.

12. In *Pathways to Madness* (New York: Vintage Books, 1973), pp. 200–203, 249–251, 313–316.

13. Ibid., p. 314. The quotation is from *Either/Or,* Vol. I (New York: Doubleday, 1959), p. 221.

14. Wolfhart Pannenberg, *Theology and the Kingdom of God* (Philadelphia: Westminster Press, 1969), p. 69.

15. See Jules Henry, *Pathways to Madness,* especially the account of "The Wilson Family."

16. See, for example, Stanley Hauerwas, "The Demands and Limits of Love: Ethical Reflections on the Moral Dilemma of Neonatal Intensive Care," and "Having and Learning How to Care for Retarded Children: Some Reflections," both included in this volume.

17. The last phrase is the title of a novel by Robert Heinlein, *Time Enough for Love* (New York: G. P. Putnam's Sons, 1974).

18. Kluge, *The Practice of Death,* (New Haven: Yale University Press, 1975), pp. 124–126.

19. Gustafson, *Theology and Christian Ethics* (Philadelphia: Pilgrim Press, 1974), p. 170.

20. This, of course, raises the larger question to what extent the language of "rights" can be used in Christian ethical discourse. For a good analysis of this problem see Joseph Allen, "A Theological Approach to Moral Rights," *The Journal of Religious Ethics,* 2, 1 (Spring, 1974), 119–141. See also my "Rights, Duties, and Experimentation on Children: A Critical Response to Worsfold and Bartholome," *Proceedings of the National Commission for Research on Human Subjects* (forthcoming).

21. Admittedly this last phrase is extremely ambiguous. We will try to give it more clarity in 3.2.

22. *The Hastings Center Report,* 5, 2 (April, 1975), 32.

23. Ibid., p. 34.

24. Ivan Illich, "The Political Uses of Natural Death," *Hastings Center Studies,* 2, 1 (January, 1974), 3–20.

25. Knud Lögstrup, *The Ethical Demand* (Philadelphia: Fortress, 1971), p. 8.

26. See Henry, *Pathways to Madness,* especially "The Jones Family."

27. See Colin Turnbull's *The Mountain People* for a frightening description of a society which is forced to abandon luxuries like trust and love. (New York: Simon and Schuster, 1972).

28. That judgmental finger might just as often be brought against the society in which the suicide lived.

29. See Yale Kamisar, "Some Non-Religious Views Against Proposed Mercy Killing Legislation," in A. B. Downing (ed.), *Euthanasia* (London: Owen, 1974), pp. 85–133.

30. Eugene Genovese, *Roll, Jordan, Roll* (New York: Pantheon Books, 1974), pp. 639–640.

31. The quotation from MacIntyre appears in his essay on "How to Identify Ethical Principles," prepared for the National Commission for the Protection of Human Subjects of Biomedical and Behavioral Research.

32. For example, see Thomas Szasz's defense of suicide as a moral category in his "The Nature of Suicide," *The Antioch Review*, 31 (Spring, 1971), 7–17.

33. G. K. Chesterton, *Orthodoxy* (London: Fontana Books, 1963), pp. 58–59.

34. See the discussion on the ethics of death in Hauerwas, *Vision and Virtue: Essays in Christian Ethical Reflection* (Notre Dame: Fides, 1974), pp. 166–186.

35. On this issue, of course, hangs much of the tragedy of the Quinlan case. For a particularly useful analysis of the ethical issues involved in that case see Paul Ramsey's, "Prolonged Dying: Not Medically Indicated," *The Hastings Center Report*, 6, 1 (February, 1976), 14–17. Ramsey argues, we think correctly, that the language of ordinary and extraordinary should be abandoned, "and that instead we should speak of (1) a comparison of treatments that are medically indicated and expected to be helpful, and those that are *not* medically indicated. In the case of the dying, that includes in all cases, or in most or many cases, a judgment that further curative treatment is no *longer* indicated. Instead of the traditional language, still current among physicians, we should talk about (2) a patient's right to refuse treatment" (p. 15). Thus, Ramsey suggests that the "treatments" given Ms. Quinlan should not be prolonged because they only act to prolong her dying. For this kind of analysis applied to those only new in life, see Hauerwas, "The Demands and Limits of Care: Ethical Reflections on the Moral Dilemma of Neonatal Intensive Care," included in this volume.

36. Oates was a member of Scott's Antarctic expedition. He had been severely injured. Knowing that the others would refuse to leave him and yet would be dangerously delayed in taking him along, he told the others he was going out for a walk and disappeared into a blizzard. R. F. Holland gives a persuasive account of why this is not suicide in his article, "Suicide," in James Raches (ed.), *Moral Problems* (New York: Harper & Row, 1971), pp. 345–359.

7: THE MORAL LIMITS OF POPULATION CONTROL

1. Quoted in Garrett Hardin (ed.), *Population, Evolution, and Birth Control* (San Francisco: W. H. Freeman and Co., 1964), pp. 77–78.

2. Barry Commoner, *The Closing Circle: Nature, Man and Technology* (New York: Alfred A. Knopf, 1971), pp. 233, 133–139.

3. Frank Notestein, "Zero Population Growth: What Is It?" in Daniel Callahan (ed.), *The American Population Debate* (New York: Anchor Books, 1971), p. 37. See also Notestein's critique of the ZPG movement in his "Zero Population Growth," *Population Index*, 36 (October–December, 1970), 444–452.

4. Ansley Coale, "Man and His Environment," in *The American Population Debate*, p. 175. A reduction in population growth gradually increases the age level of a society.

5. Many of the essays in *The American Population Debate* deal with this issue.

6. For example, in *The Report of the President's Commission on Population Growth and the American Future* it is stated: "We believe that abortion should not be considered a substitute for birth control, but rather as one element in a comprehensive system of maternal and infant health care." "Infant health care"—surely they cannot be serious to recommend abortion as a form of "infant health care." For the Commission's general discussion of abortion see pp. 172–178. Though the Commission denies it is recommending abortion as a form of population control it is at least strongly suggested by their advocacy of abortion on request.

7. William and Paul Paddock, "Today Hungry Nations, Tomorrow Starving Nations," in *The American Population Debate*, pp. 110–134.

8. *Science*, 13 (1968), 1247.

9. Paul Ehrlich, *The Population Bomb* (New York: Ballantine, 1968).

10. See for example the Club of Rome's *The Limits to Growth* (New York: Universe Books, 1972) for an attempt to set the problem in world-wide perspective. This study has been justifiably criticized for its own simplistic methodology.

11. Ben Wattenberg, "The Nonsense Explosion," in *The American Population Debate*, pp. 105–106.

12. Richard Neuhaus, *In Defense of People: Ecology and the Seduction of Radicalism* (New York: Macmillan Co., 1971), p. 114.

13. Wattenberg, p. 109.

14. This report was prepared for the President's Commission on Population Growth and the American Future. It can be obtained by writing the Hastings Center.

15. *Ethics, Population, and the American Future*, p. 15.

16. Charles Fried, *An Anatomy of Values* (Cambridge: Harvard University Press, 1970), p. 61. Fried's dependence on Rawls is evident. Even though I remain unconvinced that the "difference principle" is compatible with "equal liberty," I am convinced that something like the difference principle is a necessary condition for any society that wishes to be good.

17. Paul Ehrlich and Richard Harriman, *How To Be A Survivor* (New York: Ballantine Books, 1971), pp. 125–126, 14.

18. Paul Ehrlich, "Playboy Interview: Dr. Paul Erhlich," *Playboy Magazine* (August, 1970).

19. For an excellent article that makes this point see Arthur Dyck, "Population Policies and Ethical Acceptability," in *The American Population Debate*, pp. 351–377.

20. Martin Golding, "Obligations to Future Generations," *The Monist*, 56 (January, 1972), 85–99.

21. Daniel Callahan, "What Obligation Do We Have to Future Generations," *American Ecclesiastical Review* (April, 1971), 27.

22. Golding, p. 86.

23. Callahan, p. 23.

24. *How To Be A Survivor*, p. 14.

8:   MUST A PATIENT BE A PERSON TO BE A PATIENT?

1. Paul Ramsey, *The Patient as Person* (New Haven: Yale University Press, 1970).

2. For a more extended analysis of this point, see my *Vision and Virtue: Essays in Christian Ethical Reflection* (Notre Dame, Ind.: Fides Press, 1974).

3. Joseph Fletcher, "Indicators of Humanhood," *Hastings Center Report,* November, 1972, pp. 1-3; also see my response in "The Retarded and the Criteria of Human," included in this volume.

4. Michael Tooley, "A Defense of Abortion and Infanticide," in Joel Feinberg (ed.), *The Problem of Abortion* (Belmont: Wadsworth Publishing Co. 1973), pp. 51-91.

5. For an extended analysis of these issues, see my "The Demands and Limits of Care: Ethical Reflections on the Moral Dilemma of Neonatal Intensive Care," included in this volume.

6. Alasdair MacIntyre, "How Virtues Become Vices: Values, Medicine and Social Context," *Evaluation and Explanation in the Biomedical Sciences* (Dordrecht: Reidel, 1975), pp. 97-111.

7. For I would not deny that advocates of "person," or the regulatory notion of medical care, are right to assume that the notion of person involves the basic libertarian values of our society. It is my claim that such values are not adequate to direct medicine in a humane and/or Christian manner.

8. For an analysis of the political theory implications of my argument here see Robert Paul Wolff's, "There's Nobody Here But Us Persons," in Carol Gould and Marx Wartofsky (eds.), *Women and Philosophy: Toward a Theory of Liberation* (New York: Putnam's Sons, 1976), pp. 128-144. Wolff points out that there is a paradox of ideology in modern America.

Radical critics of American life and society attack racism, sexism, discrimination against the old, and other injustices of the public realm. They argue that the work world, and the political world, should be blind to a person's sex, or race, or age, or religion. These same critics—among whom I include myself—condemn the inhumanity of capitalism, the destruction of the human character of work, the alienation of the worker from his labor, from his product, from his fellow workers, and from his own human essence. But the very same principle of political philosophy and social organization is at work in the causes we champion and in the alienation we condemn. To ignore the sex, race, age, culture, religion, or personality of a person when hiring, or paying, or electing, or admitting that person, is to accept the public-private split, and to shove into the private sphere, out of sight and out of consideration, everything that makes a person a human being and not merely a rational agent. I am not a person who just happens, accidently and irrelevantly, to be a man, forty years old, the husband of a professor of English literature, the son of two aging and sick parents, the father of two small boys six and four, a comfortable well-off member of the upper-middle class, American-Jewish born and raised in New York. I am *essentially* such a man. . . . To demand that the public world of work and politics be blind to age, sex, race, and so forth precisely *is* to equate the most essential facts of my human self with relatively trivial facts of my tastes and preferences, and to consign them all to the private world where they will have no influence on *important* public policies and decisions (pp. 136-137).

9: THE POLITICS OF CHARITY

1. It may be that this is the only safe generalization that can be made about "liberation theology." For "liberation theology" is currently used to identify every movement that claims to be for man and against oppression. Because of this it is extremely

difficult to separate the various claims and issues associated with this style of theology. For an attempt, however, to analyze how the claims of "political theology" may differ from "liberation theology" see Francis Fiorenza's "Political Theology and Liberation Theology: An Inquiry Into Their Fundamental Meaning," in *Liberation, Revolution, and Freedom: Theological Perspectives* (New York: Seabury Press, 1975), pp. 3–29. For a good anthology that illustrates how different the interests of "political theology" are from liberation theology see Jurgen Moltmann et al., *Religion and Political Society*, (New York: Harper & Row, 1974). For example, the overriding concern of the "political theologian" with the problems of the enlightenment in contrast to the "theology of liberation" is strikingly obvious from the essays in this volume. As will be clear from this essay, I am generally unsympathetic with the manner that "liberation theology" tries to form the issue of how Christians have a political responsibility to serve the poor. This is especially the case, as many times advocates of this position tend to confuse political freedom with that offered by Christ. However, for a very substantial and insightful articulation of a "political theology," see William Coats, *God in Public: Political Theology Beyond Niebuhr* (Grand Rapids: Eerdmans, 1974). Coats rightly emphasizes the value of equality rather than freedom as the overriding social virtue. Paradoxically, most writers in liberation theology have failed to see that the emphasis on freedom as the pre-emptory value of the political order continues to presuppose the libertarian society that has created the inequalities they feel so strongly about.

2. The relationship between Niebuhr and liberation theology would make a study in itself. Most of the liberation theologians want, like Niebuhr, to warrant the use of power and force by Christians to overthrow what they consider unjust social orders. But theologians of liberation do not share Niebuhr's sober realism about the limits of the good such action can accomplish. In Niebuhr's terms the theologians of liberation are the "children of light" who fail to see that the attempt to do good can at best only produce a lesser evil. For Niebuhr's analysis of the children of light see his *The Children of Light and the Children of Darkness*, (New York: Charles Scribner's Sons, 1944). I am sympathetic with the theologians of liberation dissatisfaction with Niebuhr- ian realism. However, my dissatisfaction is more with Niebuhr's failure to see that his own analysis of the limits of political action indicates that there are limits to what Christians can do in the interest of building the good society. For further reflections along this line see my "The Future of Christian Social Ethics," in George Devine (ed.), *That They May Live* (New York: Alba House, 1972), pp. 123–131.

3. Quoted by Paul Lehmann in his *The Transfiguration of Politics* (New York: Harper and Row, 1975). See also my review of Lehmann's book in *Worldview* 18, 12 (December, 1975), 45–48.

There are a number of interesting things about this quote that would require exten- sive analysis to treat adequately. However, it should at least be noted that Torres simply assumes that the dissatisfaction of the majority constituted sufficient justifica- tion for revolution. Even if one ignores the problem raised by majoritarian democracy, it still remains to be shown how the democratic model can be harmonized with the totalitarian organizations necessary for successful revolutionary activity. See for example my "Democracy as the Quest for Legitimate Authority," *The Review of Politics*, 34, 1 (January, 1972), 117–124. Secondly, Torres assumes that the love required of Christians is directed at all people. However, such a love is presumptive as well as being destructive because it must end by justifying the coercion of some for the good of the greater number. As I will try to show, the Christian is obligated to love his neighbor, not all men. The significance of the Gospel involves how it gives us the skill to patiently love and care for some when not all can be loved and cared for. Put differently, the primary political contribution of the Gospel is not to tell us that we ought to love our neighbor, but rather how such love should be formed in a world where the good must be done even though tragedy surrounds it.

4. See, for example, John Howard Yoder's, *The Politics of Jesus* (Grand Rapids: Eerdmans, 1973) and my essay on Yoder, "Messianic Pacifism," *Worldview*, 16, 6 (June, 1973), 29–33.

5. See John Howard Yoder's critique of the way liberation theologians tend to confuse the "poor" with the people of God in his "Exodus and Exile: The Two Faces of Liberation," *Cross Currents*, 23 (1973), 297–309.

6. Richard Schaull, "Revolutionary Change in Theological Perspective," in Gibson Winter (ed.), *Social Ethics* (New York: Harper and Row, 1968), pp. 234–235.

7. Albert Camus, *The Rebel: An Essay on Man in Revolt* (New York: Vintage, 1956), p. 25. Moreover, Schaull, like many theologians of liberation, fails to distinguish political revolution from social revolution. What they clearly care about is social revolution, but they talk as if shifting the power relations in a society at the level of the state can bring about the kind of society they want. But everything we know about the history of revolutions tends to deny that it is possible without forming a totalitarian government to affect deeply the form of a social order by changing those that rule. Mao, of course, is the primary example of what can be done if you are willing to give up on the value of freedom.

8. The issue of the authority and how scripture is to be used in ethical reflection is a complex and confused subject at present in theological ethics. It is my hope that the way I have used scripture will at least suggest one way that scripture can be used to illuminate ethical reflection. For a more systematic analysis of this issue see James Gustafson, *Theology and Christian Ethics* (Philadelphia: Pilgrim Press, 1974), pp. 121–160.

9. For the interpretation of Luke presented here I am primarily indebted to Hans Conzelmann's *The Theology of St. Luke* (London: Faber and Faber, 1960); and Jacob Jervell, *Luke and the People of God* (Minneapolis: Aubsburg Publishing House, 1972).

10. For further reflections on this theme see my "Natural Law, Tragedy, and Theological Ethics" included in this volume.

11. Julius Lester suggests,

When a people choose to define themselves as oppressed, they choose to live by the world's definitions. And when theology speaks in the language of the world and seeks to merge itself with the world's definitions, it has become an instrument of the very oppression it claims to oppose. . . . We are called upon to be saints. That is the message of the Sermon on the Mount. In it Jesus speaks with terrifying simplicity: "Be ye therefore perfect, even as your Father which is in Heaven is perfect." Is that what frightens us? Is that why we try to recruit God to lead the revolutionary vanguard and join the women's movement? Is that why we get all tangled up in eschatologies and apocalypses? Is it because Jesus told us in the most simple, straightforward language ever used what it is we are to do with our lives? "But that's hard, Jesus. Be Perfect? Hey, man! Lighten up! It's easier to be Black, white, male, female, a theologian, man, than to be perfect like God." But that is precisely what Jesus said: "Be ye therefore perfect." And he wouldn't have said it if it wasn't possible ("Be ye therefore perfect," *Kattallagete* [Winter, 1974], pp. 25, 27).

Implied in Lester's remarks is the claim that the most radical political action the church can perform is to provide the symbolic categories that help free us from the world's description of what constitutes freedom. We forget that part of the power of the political is the power of the description of what is going on.

12. Hannah Arendt, for example, has argued that violence occurs when a people no longer have the power to act in common—that is, when they have no shared symbols that they hold as true. *On Violence* (New York: Harcourt, Brace, and World, 1969), pp. 44–56.

13. For a perspective very similar to this see Hannah Arendt, "Truth and Politics," in Peter Laslett and W. G. Runciman (eds.), *Philosophy, Politics, and Society,* Third Series (Oxford: Basil Blackwell, 1967). Ms. Arendt argues that

> as far as action is concerned, organized lying is a marginal phenomenon, but the trouble is that its opposite, the mere telling of facts, leads to no action whatsoever. It even tends, under normal circumstances, to accept things as they are. Truthfulness has never been counted among the political virtues because it has indeed little to contribute to that change of world and circumstances which is among the most legitimate political activities. Only when a community has embarked upon organized lying on principle, and not only with respect to particulars, can truthfulness as such, unsupported by the distorting forces of power and interest, become a political factor of the first order. Where everybody lies about everything of importance, the truth teller, whether he knows it or not, has begun to act, he too has engaged himself in political business; for in the unlikely event that he survives, he has started to change the world (p. 123).

Ms. Arendt points out that the lie in politics is especially resistant to the truth for the very loyalty of people to the lie gives it the form of truth. The more successful liar is exactly the one that is most likely to fall prey, therefore, to his own fabrications. Thus the problem of truth in politics is more complicated because lies are seldom blatant but the half-truth of self-deception. What is needed, if a polity is to even begin to approach the truth, is a people who are formed by a story that gives them the skills not to fear the truth. For more on this see my and David Burrell's, "Self-Deception and Autobiography: Theological and Ethical Reflections on Speer's *Inside the Third Reich,*" included in this volume.

14. I am, of course, thinking of John Rawls, *A Theory of Justice* (Cambridge: Harvard University Press, 1971), and Robert Nozick's *Anarchy, State, and Utopia* (New York: Basic Books, 1975).

15. Rawls and Nozick in quite different ways have a conception of the good but interpret it in strong, individualistic terms. The good I am suggesting is those forms of life a people have come to share that provide a center of loyalty from which the individual learns what it means to be moral. Rawls and Nozick are trying to provide a political ethic for a society of strangers, but I remain unconvinced that any such account can do justice to the form of community necessary for the good society. Finally, there is no way to avoid the question of what kind of virtues citizens should have if the good society is to be realized.

10: HAVING AND LEARNING TO CARE FOR RETARDED CHILDREN

1. *St. Anthony Messenger,* June, 1975, p. 4.

2. For example see my "The Family: Theological and Ethical Reflections," in Van Kussrow and Richard Baepler (eds.), *Changing American Life Styles* (Valparaiso: University of Valparaiso Press, 1977), pp. 111–119.

3. In the absence of any reason to have children the language of the "rights of children" has been used to try to protect children from their parents and society. Such language, however, only reinforces societal assumptions that make the family appear irrational or even absurd. In this respect see my "Rights, Duties, and the Experimentation on Children: A Critical Response to Worsfold and Bartholome," *Proceedings of the National Commission for Research on Human Subjects* (forthcoming).

4. Milton Mayerhoff, *On Caring* (New York: Harper & Row, 1971), p. 1.

13: THE DEMANDS AND LIMITS OF CARE

1. *Time*, March 25, 1974, p. 84. For a similar article see "Shall This Child Die," *Newsweek*, March 12, 1973, p. 70.

2. For an extended discussion and defense of these claims see my *Vision and Virtue: Essays in Christian Ethical Reflection* (Notre Dame, Ind.: Fides Press, 1974).

3. Herbert Fingarette, *Self Deception* (New York: Humanities Press, 1969); see also David Burrell and Stanley Hauerwas, "Self-Deception and Autobiography: Theological and Ethical Reflections on Speer's *Inside the Third Reich,*" included in this volume.

4. The moral context in which we must do ethical reflection is another reason we must begin with this more basic question. For to be able to give a direct answer to the question, "What should we do?" assumes a moral community and consensus that simply is not present. As Paul Ramsey has suggested,

> Ethical inquiry and discourse begin only when we discover we are in disagreement about what we ought to do. Then we are forced back upon our premises, and we must seek together in the human community and in the medical profession to find agreement at a deeper level. We must ask about what makes anything right. We need to find out if we can agree upon the right-making or wrong-making features of moral attitudes, actions, roles or relations, before returning to the specific case where we first disagreed over what ought to be done. This is ethics proper. It is also why in any age every moral agent is an ethicist if he will only let himself go and be one; and why in a period in which there is a moral consensus, ethics mainly gives backing to the consensus and few are needed for that important function. In any age, however, when ancient landmarks have been removed, and we are trying to do the unthinkable, namely build a civilization without an agreed civil tradition and upon the absence of a moral consensus, everyone needs to be an ethicist to the extent of his capacity for reflection and his desire to be and to know that he is a responsible person ("The Nature of Medical Ethics" in R. M. Veatch, W. Gaylin, and C. Morgan [eds.], *The Teaching of Medical Ethics* [Hastings, New York: A Hastings Center Publication, 1973], p. 15).

5. Mary Douglas, *Purity and Danger: An Analysis of Concepts of Pollution and Taboo* (London: Rutledge and Kegan Paul, 1966), p. 39.

6. John Fletcher, "Attitudes Toward Defective Newborns," *Hastings Center Studies,* 2, 1 (January, 1974), 23.

7. Ramsey argues, "We would not be able to determine the appropriate decision maker if we had no notion of the appropriate decision to be made. Absent any normative ethics on the urgent moral question we face, however, and inevitably deciding-who-shall-decide becomes a substitute for ethical inquiry and discourse about what

ought to be done (whoever does it)." "The Nature of Medical Ethics," p. 18. It may be in cases of extreme ambiguity the question of "Who" becomes more important as it seems just that those who will bear the burden of the decision should make it.

8. Fletcher provides a good account of the almost universal negative reaction parents feel on the birth of a defective newborn. "Attitudes Toward Defective Newborns," pp. 24–32.

9. James Gustafson provides an excellent analysis of the parents' and physicians' points of view in "Mongolism, Parental Desires, and the Right to Life," *Perspective in Biology and Medicine*, 16, 4 (Summer, 1973), 539–548.

10. This is the main moral issue raised by Duff and Campbell as they recommend doctors give parents the alternative not to care for their child. This may be a good thing, but it significantly changes the morality of the case. Unfortunately Duff and Campbell give no criteria to determine when the doctor should describe the case in this manner and when he should not. Thus they give no ethical criteria that might act as a guide to how defective a newborn must be for this kind of alternative to be given to parents. Raymond Duff and A. G. M. Campbell, "Moral and Ethical Dilemmas in the Special-Care Nursery," *The New England Journal of Medicine*, 289, 17 (October 24, 1973).

11. In a letter to the *Washington Post* Fred Carney rightly argues that these cases should not be left to the arbitrary judgments of either parents or doctors no matter how altruistic they may be.

What is obviously needed is the development of substantive standards to inform parents and physicians who must make such decisions. The professional inputs of physicians, ethicists, social workers, lawyers and others should be involved in formulating them. My own beliefs about the content of such standards are that they should grant primacy to the interest of the baby, that they should not include individually-varying social circumstances in the assessment of a baby's interest, and that it be considered in the baby's interest to let him die only when deformity is so disastrous as to place him in a category upon which there is general medical agreement that the physiological potential for meaningful life is utterly missing. My own beliefs on these matters aside, it is urgent that society encourage the development of substantive standards for protecting the interest of deformed babies, indeed, that society direct more of its attention and resources generally to the critical assessment of ethical issues in biological and other aspects of public policy (Wednesday, March 20, 1974, p. A. 15).

12. Joseph Fletcher is perhaps the clearest exponent of this position. See his "Indicators of Humanhood," *The Hastings Center Report* (November, 1972), pp. 1–3 and my response "The Retarded and the Criteria of the Human," included in this volume.

13. Duff and Campbell, "Moral and Ethical Dilemmas in the Special-Care Nursery," p. 893. One of the most disturbing aspects of some of the literature dealing with these issues is the use of jargon. In a period when our political institutions have been corrupted by describing burglary as surreptitious entry it would seem that we would be more sensitive than to describe death as a "management option." The main thrust of this essay is that as crucial as what we decide about these cases is the kind of language we should learn to use about them.

14. For some this may seem an extremely odd or even immoral question, yet it can be asked by the most humane person. I suspect what causes us to deny the humanity of another is not our insensitivity, though that is often the case, but our sensitivity. The one that suffers somehow seems less threatening if we see him as less than our own

kind. For example, this may be the reason doctors often appear so professionally distant and thus let themselves be open to the charge of acting impersonally. For how much suffering can you stand to be around without it perverting the soul? The doctor's impersonal professionalism is absolutely necessary if he is able to continue to feel at all. It is a way of blocking out the constant suffering around him, so that he might still respond to suffering in selected cases.

15. It is impossible to develop this complex issue beyond these brief remarks, as it involves the whole question of human embodiment. For a good analysis of these issues see H. Tristram Engelhardt, "The Process of Embodiment and Bioethics," unpublished paper (Galveston, Texas: University of Texas Medical School). I have great sympathy with Professor Engelhardt's critique of dualist and monistic models of the self; however, I do not think his ethical conclusions necessarily follow from his analysis of human ontogeny. Michael Tooley has provided the most extended argument for distinguishing "persons" as possessors of rights from being a member of the human species. Tooley thus willingly defends infanticide, as the infant, even though a member of the human species, has none of the characteristics we associate with being a person. "A Defense of Abortion and Infanticide," in Joel Feinberg (ed.), *The Problem of Abortion* (Belmont: Wadsworth Publishing Co., 1973), pp. 51–91. S. I. Benn argues against Tooley that there may be relevant reasons against infanticide that are not based on the "right to life."

16. Duff and Campbell in a bizarre manner turn the language of right to life against itself and suggest that they are simply affording these children the "right to die." "Moral and Ethical Dilemmas in the Special-Care Nursery," p. 892. Such a suggestion fails entirely to note the difference, even if there is such a thing as the "right to die," between exercising that right for oneself and having it exercised for you such as it is in these cases. Moreover, if these children are not persons, as Duff and Campbell seem to suggest, then it is unclear if rights language is applicable to them at all, whether it be the right to life or death. Generally it should be pointed out that the very idea of a "right to life" is problematic, for it is unclear on what basis anyone might be able to make such a claim. It may well be that inasmuch as any of us have rights we have a right not to be put to death, but that is quite different from the idea that all men have something like an absolute right to life.

17. Engelhardt argues that "rights are those values which persons can claim as their own. Only persons have rights and that they have them is in virtue of the claim which they themselves make. Only persons are self-conscious, and therefore conscious of their value, and therefore free to claim it. The possession of value involved in rights presupposes an element of self-conscious, rational thought, without which there would be an inclination towards but not a claiming of a value." "The Process of Embodiment and Bioethics," p. 13. Engelhardt's argument is shared by many philosophers, as it is assumed that characteristics that persons must have to have rights at least must involve the ability to make known their basic interests. See, for example, Henry David Aiken's, "Life and the Right to Life," in B. Hilton, D. Callahan, M. Harris, P. Condliffe, and B. Berkley (eds.), *Ethical Issues in Human Genetics* (New York: Plenum Press, 1973), pp. 173–183. Joel Feinberg offers a more generous account by arguing that logically all that is necessary for a being to have rights is that they have interests—that is that they are capable of being harmed or benefited. See his "The Rights of Animals and Future Generations," paper delivered at the University of Notre Dame.

I cannot possibly try to unravel all that is involved in the issue of what moral psychology must be presupposed to make sense of rights. However, a theological analysis of rights language might provide an alternative account. For as Joseph Allen points out, theologically the recognition of the worth of a person

> is inseparably connected with being a person created by God. This faith provides no basis for asserting that children are without rights, any more than are the ignorant, the weak, or the alien. The problem still remains what are the various characteristics that must be present before one must be called a person, and thus be deemed to have the kinds of rights that persons have ... does one become a person, and thus of worth individually as an end, at conception, or implantation, or some later point in development before birth, or at birth, or sometime afterward? Plausible answers to that questions from a Christian perspective will hinge upon the identification of those characteristics essential to being a person. The point here is that from the standpoint of Christian faith one would resist the temptation to identify the essential characteristics of personhood in such a way as to create a weapon with which one's own social or cultural group might oppress another. Whatever physical-psychological prerequisites there are for personhood, or for its potentiality, all who have these without exclusion, are individually of worth as ends ("A Theological Approach to Moral Rights," *Journal of Religious Ethics*, II, 119–139).

18. Engelhardt, for example, argues children may be bearers of social value.
19. Hauerwas, "The Retarded and the Criteria of the Human."
20. G. J. Warnock, *The Object of Morality* (London: Methuen, 1971), p. 151.
21. Peter Singer, "Animal Liberation," *New York Review of Books*, 20, 5 (April 15, 1973), 17. Of course the question remains what kind of beings are capable of suffering. Singer argues that this does not depend on verbal skills, or self-reflection, but the ability to gesture appropriate behavioral signs.
22. Ivan Illich argues that our sense of "natural death" has been transformed by medicine's ability to create new expectations of health. "The Political Uses of Natural Death," *The Hastings Center Studies*, 2, 1 (January, 1974), 3–20. This issue involves the attempt to distinguish between ordinary and extraordinary means to save life. It seems doubtful if this distinction can be saved from the ambiguities surrounding it. However, for a good analysis of the distinction, see Paul Ramsey's *The Patient as Person* (New Haven: Yale University Press, 1970), pp. 118–124.
23. The significance of the methodological assumptions underlying this essay is perhaps most clearly seen in this context. For my difficulty with both a consequential and formal ethical analysis is the tendency to abstract the case from the agents and roles that form the situation. I suspect that this is always a tendency in an ethics of obligation where one is more concerned with an external observer's judgment about the action. As Carney has made clear, any adequate account of the moral life must combine virtue and obligation notions. "The Virtue-Obligation Controversy," *Journal of Religious Ethics*, 1 (Fall, 1973), 5–19. See also in the same issue my "The Self as Story: Religion and Morality from the Agent's Perspective," pp. 73–85. Put concretely, the proper ethical question concerning these cases is not, "What should we do?" but rather "What kind of parent should I be to be able to welcome a defective child into this world in a humane and caring manner?"
24. For a very perceptive article on current American attitudes about having children see Garry Wills, "What? What? Are Young Americans Afraid to Have Kids?" *Esquire*, 81, 3 (March, 1974), 80, 170–172.
25. Sumner Twiss provides an excellent discussion of the issues raised concerning parental duty to avoid bearing children with serious genetic defects. "Parental Responsibility for Genetic Health," *The Hastings Center Report*, 4, 1 (February, 1974),

9-11. Of course I am not denying that it is a good thing if possible to take precautions that might prevent genetic birth defects. I am simply suggesting that our obligation as parents does not include assuring our children perfect physical existence.

26. The larger issue, of course, is whether happiness is an adequate metaphor for the moral life. As Bernard Williams observes, "The views of certain philosophers of antiquity, that virtue was sufficient for happiness and that the good man could be happy on the rack, have been rightly thought before, after, and no doubt during their time to involve some paradox. But if happiness is ultimately incompatible with too much, or too total, suffering, there can perhaps be recognizably moral outlooks which reject the notion that happiness is the concern of our arrangements." Williams goes on to suggest that "Men do, as a matter of fact, find value in such things as submission, trust, uncertainty, risk, even despair and suffering, and these values can scarcely all be related to a central idea of *happiness*." Bernard Williams, *Morality: An Introduction to Ethics* (New York: Harper and Row, 1972), pp. 82, 87. For a similar position see my "Love Is Not All You Need," in *Vision and Virtue*. In the context of this issue I think the formalists are completely right.

27. Hal Moore, "Acting and Refraining," unpublished manuscript (U. of Notre Dame). I am not suggesting that action must be conscious in order to be an action, but rather that if conscious action is the paradigm instance of action then clearly refraining is action. See also Jonathan Bennett's, "Whatever the Consequences," in James Rachels (ed.), *Moral Problems* (New York: Harper and Row, 1971), pp. 43–66.

28. This also has implications for interpreting the doctrine of double effect, but to raise this issue would take us beyond the scope of this paper. For a recent discussion of the doctrine of double effect see Richard McCormick, *Ambiguity in Moral Choice* (Milwaukee: Marquette University, 1973).

29. I am relying here on Philippa Foot's argument in her "The Problem of Abortion and the Doctrine of the Double Effect," in Rachels, pp. 29–41. For a similar discussion see Jeffrie Murphey, "The Killing of the Innocent," *The Monist*, 57, 4 (October, 1973), 527–550. There is obviously a good deal of ambiguity in trying to draw a hard and fast line between positive and negative obligation. However, I do not think that the ambiguity of certain cases destroys the general intent of the distinction. However, for a counter argument, see Tooley, "A Defense of Abortion and Infanticide," pp. 84–85.

30. John Casey, "Actions and Consequences," in *Morality and Moral Reasoning* (London: Methuen, 1971), p. 168.

31. Moreover this raises the question of who should do the killing or if you prefer in whose presence the child should "be let die." It may be that parents may have the right to refuse care for their children, but they do not have the right to ask doctors to bear the consequences of the decision, nor should doctors accept such responsibility if it is the nurses who must actually bear the burden of caring for the child.

32. For a more extended discussion of this point see my "The Ethics of Death: Letting Die or Putting to Death," *Vision and Virtue*.

33. An excellent discussion of the moral issues involved in the question of the meaning of health can be found in "The Concept of Health," *Hastings Center Studies*, 1, 3 (1973).

34. Ramsey, "The Nature of Medical Ethics," p. 24. For a more extended discussion by Ramsey of this distinction see his *Patient as Person* (New Haven: Yale University Press, 1970), pp. 113–164.

35. It is instructive to note the significance in this respect of the religious sense in seeing children as "gifts from God." For the grammar of "gift" implies that the child

is not the parents' creation, but comes as a bearer of value independent of the parents' attitudes toward the child. Moreover it makes clear that our reasons for having children are important as our reasons set the context of care. For Christians the ultimate reason for having children is that they are obligated to people the church. For a more strictly theological approach to these issues see my "Christian Care of the Retarded," *Theology Today,* 30, 2 (July, 1973), 130–137.

14: MEDICINE AS A TRAGIC PROFESSION

1. Alasdair MacIntyre, "How Virtues Become Vices: Values, Medicine and Social Context," in H. Tristram Engelhardt and Stuart Spicker (eds.), *Evaluation and Explanation in the Biomedical Sciences* (Dordrecht: D. Reidel Publishing Co., 1975), pp. 110–111. In a somewhat similar vein John Ladd has pointed out that contemporary liberal ethical theory has no place for the category of tragedy as all problems are seen either as a problem of prioritizing or a problem of the conflict of interest. As a result, liberal ethical theory cannot account for the radical sense of evil that denies "the goodness of what is good and the evilness of what is evil." "Are Science and Ethics Compatible?" in H. Tristram Engelhardt, Jr., and Daniel Callahan (eds.), *Science, Ethics, and Medicine,* I (Hastings-on-Hudson: Hastings Center Publication, 1976), 53–57.

2. For example, Eric Cassell argues that "medicine is basically a moral profession—or moral-technical, if you wish, based on the fact that physicians are directly concerned with the immediate welfare of other humans." "Moral Thought in Clinical Practice: Applying the Abstract to the Usual," in Engelhardt and Callahan, *Science, Ethics, and Medicine,* I, 150.

3. See, for example, H. Tristram Engelhardt, Jr., "The Concept of Health and Disease," in Engelhardt and Spicker, *Evaluation and Explanation . . .* , pp. 125–142; and the essays in the issue, "The Concept of Health," *Hastings Center Studies,* 1, 3 (1973).

4. Ivan Illich, *Medical Nemesis* (New York: Pantheon Books, 1976), p. 128.

5. Paul Ramsey, *Patient as Person* (New Haven: Yale University Press, 1970). For Ramsey's concern about the ethos supporting the commitment of the physician to the patient, see his "The Nature of Medical Ethics," in R. M. Veatch, W. Gaylin and C. Morgan (eds.), *The Teaching of Medical Ethics* (Hastings-on-Hudson: Hastings Center Publications, 1973), pp. 14–27; and "Conceptual Foundations for the Ethics of Medical Care: A Response," in R. M. Veatch and Roy Branson (eds.), *Ethics and Health Policy* (Cambridge: Ballinger Publishing Co., 1976), pp. 35–55. Paul Camenisch has demonstrated conclusively that for Ramsey the "concern for the individual, his integrity and his rights is a crucial driving force in his ethics; that this concern extensively shapes the task Ramsey sets for himself—that of protecting the individual, largely through the shaping and maintaining of a livable ethos; and that this concern and this task are the absolutely necessary starting points for understanding Ramsey's methodology." And further, "Ramsey is exceedingly concerned about protecting the individual from society, for Ramsey's asserting the existence of covenants and claims independently of any human willing of them almost always occurs in those biomedical contexts where such covenants and claims serve to assure the individual adequate care and to protect him from societal encroachments." "Paul Ramsey's Task: Some Meth-

odological Clarifications and Questions," James Johnson and David Smith (eds.), *"Love and Society," Essays in the Ethics of Paul Ramsey* (Missoula: Scholars Press, 1974), pp. 71, 73.

6. For an extensive argument in support of this claim see David Burrell and my, "From System to Story: An Alternative Pattern for Rationality in Ethics," an essay included in the present volume. My use of "narrative" and "story" in this essay obviously has a technical meaning I cannot analyze here. However, see the above for an attempt to spell out the significance of these terms.

7. Illich, *Medical Nemesis*, p. 9.

8. Ibid., p. 30.

9. Ibid., pp. 127, 133.

10. For a good analysis of the difference between "rationalist" and "empiric" views of medicine see Lester King, "Values in Medicine," in Engelhardt and Callahan, *Science, Ethics, and Medicine*, I, 233–234. King demonstrates that "the values of medical practice are distinct from the values in medical theory," in the sense that we may often be giving better care than we have the theoretical means to account for. This causes no great difficulty for the practice of medicine except that it causes confusion, particularly in matters of medical ethics, as the physician may often misdescribe what in fact he is doing. What this suggests is that much of the task of medical ethics is simply trying to help the physician say what morally he is doing. If we lack an adequate language the danger is that the language we in fact do use will be seized by a different kind of story that is all the more powerful because we do not recognize that it has us in its power.

11. Lewis Thomas, "Rx for Illich," *New York Review of Books*, 23, 14 (September 16, 1976), 3.

12. Ernest Becker, *The Structure of Evil* (New York: Braziller, 1968), p. 18.

13. Thomas, "Rx for Illich," p. 4.

14. Ibid. In a like manner Eric Cassell says, "Life is the problem—providing meaning and fulfillment, depth and happiness in life. These tasks, requiring a whole lifetime, are beyond the function of the physician. It is true that he can make the job of living harder by maintaining fear of the body and fear of death. And he can make the job easier by teaching how to live with the body, how to surmount illness and conquer disability. Creating happiness is not the work of the physician. That task must be achieved by each of us alone, as it always has been." *The Healer's Art* (New York: Lippincott, 1976), p. 182. What neither Thomas nor Cassell indicates, however, is what kind of ethos will sustain medicine that does not try to free us from the fated aspects of our existence.

15. For a useful discussion of the meaning of profession see Wilbert Moore, *The Profession: Roles and Rules* (New York: Russell Sage Foundation, 1970). Moore thinks that definitions of professions have little value because the attributes of the persons taken to be professionals may have only an approximate fit with persons identified as professionals by others. He therefore suggests that characteristics of the professions be seen as a scale along which many different kinds can fit. He thus proposes the following characteristics,

The professional practices a full-time occupation, which comprises the principal source of his earned income. . . . A more distinctively professional qualification is that of commitment to a calling, that is, the treatment of the occupation and all its requirements as an enduring set of normative and behavioral expectations. Those who pursue occupations of relatively high rank in terms of criteria of professionalism are likely to be set apart from the laity by various signs and symbols, but by the same token are identified with their peers—often in formalized organizations. . . . An important next step in professionalism is the possession of esoteric but useful knowledge and skills, based on specialized training or education of exceptional duration and perhaps of exceptional difficulty. The qualification "useful" knowledge implies the next higher scale position of professionalism: in the practice of his occupation, the professional is expected to exhibit a service orientation, to perceive the needs of individual or collective clients that are relevant to his competence and to attend to those needs by competent performance. Finally, in the use of his exceptional knowledge, the professional proceeds by his own judgment and authority; he thus enjoys autonomy restrained by responsibility (pp. 5–6).

16. Stephen Toulmin, "The Meaning of Professionalism: Doctor's Ethics and Biomedical Science," in H. Tristram Engelhardt and Daniel Callahan (eds.), *Knowledge, Value, and Belief*, II (Hastings-on-Hudson: Hastings Center Publication, 1977), 2 (in mimeograph).

17. Richard Wasserstrom, "Lawyers as Professionals: Some Moral Issues," *Human Rights*, 5 (1975), 2.

18. Ibid., p. 2.

19. John Ladd makes a useful distinction between contingent and logical incompatibility relevant to my argument. "Generally, contingent incompatibility obtains when two states of affairs (or actions) that are desired or desirable cannot, for contingent reasons, coexist. . . . Logical incompatibility, on the other hand, holds between the assertion of a value and the denial of that value." "Are Science and Ethics Compatible?" in Engelhardt and Callahan, *Science, Ethics, and Medicine*, I, p. 57. Ladd argues rightly that logical incompatibility cannot be derived from contingent incompatibility—that for some reason I cannot do my duty does not imply that it was not my duty. For example, the fact that there may be contingent incompatibility between being able to save a life and telling the truth does not mean that one of them is any less my duty, as some recent moralists have argued (Hare). I may have both duties, one of which I tragically cannot fulfill. A profession may involve incompatible duties all of which are necessary for the moral direction of the profession.

20. I am purposely leaving the sense of tragedy ambiguous as there are various kinds of "tragedies" involved in medicine. I think this is not unwarranted as the literature surrounding the question, "What is a tragedy?" demonstrates well that "tragedy" has no one meaning. Indeed it seems that those who wish to try to pin down tragedy, do so by making one play or novel paradigmatic for all others—thus *Oedipus* becomes tragedy and *Antigone* melodrama. Some philosophical formulations of the meaning of tragedy only confuse the issue further by arguing that one meaning of tragedy is more conceptually satisfying than another. This generates even more confusing discussions such as whether Christianity does not necessarily deny the existence of tragedy. For example, see D. D. Raphael, *The Paradox of Tragedy* (Bloomington: Indiana University Press, 1960).

This does not deny that it is important to distinguish between accidents, unfortunate occurrences, and tragedy. However, the ability to make such distinctions is not correlative of any one sense of tragedy, but rather depends on seeing how certain "events" fit into a narrative context. For example, I suggest that the tragic aspect of medicine involves a conflict of goods or evils and a lack of resources, but such conflicts and scarcity are but reminders that we exist in a situation that our very awareness makes more anguishing. Our temptation is to lie to ourselves and others about our situation but such a strategy only results in deepening our capacity for evil and unnecessary tragedies. It is the tragic irony of life that in the name of saving ourselves we seek our own annihilation, or destruction of the things that make our lives worthwhile. For a very helpful discussion of tragedy see Clifford Leech, *Tragedy* (London: Methuen, 1969); and for a discussion that represents the kind of analysis characteristic of literary criticism see Robert Heilman, *The Iceman, the Arsonist, and the Troubled Agent: Tragedy and Melodrama on the Modern Stage* (Seattle: University of Washington Press, 1973). I wish to thank Professor Robert King of DePaul University for helping me clarify these matters.

21. Monroe Freedman, *Lawyers' Ethics in an Adversary System* (New York: Bobbs-Merrill Co., 1975).

22. Toulmin, "The Meaning of Professionalism..." in Engelhardt and Callahan, *Knowledge, Value, and Belief,* II, 10.

23. Ibid., pp. 24–25.

24. Lester King, "Values in Medicine," in Engelhardt and Callahan, *Science, Ethics, and Medicine,* I, 232.

25. Toulmin, "The Meaning of Professionalism..." in Engelhardt and Callahan, *Knowledge, Value, and Belief,* II, 19.

26. Albert Jonsen and Andre Hellegers, "Conceptual Foundations for an Ethics of Medical Care," in Veatch and Branson, *Ethics and Health Policy,* pp. 3–20. Jonsen and Hellegers argue that any adequate medical ethics must involve a theory of virtue, a theory of duties, and a theory of the common good. Ramsey rightly criticizes them for failing to indicate that there must be some prioritizing or lexical ordering between these different aspects of the moral commitments of a physician. Ramsey argues that "there are sound grounds for saying that rules of practice or regulative 'moral notions' should be accorded priority over an ethics of doing the most good on the whole, if there are cases of irresolvable conflict between them." "Conceptual Foundations for an Ethics of Medical Care: A Response," in Veatch and Branson, *Ethics and Health Policy,* p. 49. While I think that Ramsey is right in this respect, he fails to see that the alternative is not between "rules of practice" and the "common good," as if both those were given. What must be recognized is that the doctor's commitment to his patient rests on a sense of the kind of faithfulness that makes good communities. The "rule" is not separable from the "good," but rather each is an abstraction that denotes the way a tradition has learned to value certain kinds of special relations. Our difficulty is that we have no moral theory that adequately expresses the kind of convictions that guide our lives in this respect. As a result, it looks like we choose between an ethics of "rules" or one of the "common good," when in fact the tradition holds them both. Indeed, it is the virtue of traditions to keep in tension that which cannot be resolved in theory. What is required is not a theory that effects a resolution, but a story that helps us to learn to live and to pay the price for maintaining the necessary tension.

27. MacIntyre, "How Virtues Become Vices..." in Engelhardt and Spicker, *Evaluation and Explanation,* p. 109.

28. Wasserstrom, "Lawyers as Professionals..." p. 3.

29. Ibid., p. 4. There is a normative claim underlying this analogy that I cannnot defend here. This analogy presupposes that the kind of relation between physician and patient is more like that between friend and friend than between stranger and stranger. Thus the obligations incumbent on the physician are not aspects of a general obligation we owe to all, but more like obligations that derive from special relations. Indeed, I suspect part of the problem with medical ethics has been the assumption that the language of "universal obligation" is adequate to characterize the moral convictions characteristic of medicine. Because of this we have failed to notice that medicine requires a substantive narrative to sustain the tragic implications of fulfilling our particularistically

dependent obligations. For a more systematic treatment of the kind of relationship I am suggesting as normative between doctor and patient see Charles Fried, *Medical Experimentation* (New York: American Elsevier, 1974), pp. 67–78. Fried points out that Kantian moral theory has been unable to account for personal loyalties and obligations that are the essence of the doctor-patient relation. Put in my terms, it has been the error of recent medical ethics to try to characterize the kind of obligations involved between physician and patient as if they were not dependent on a narrative context. Fried has also applied this point to the law in his "The Lawyer or Friend: The Moral Foundation of the Lawyer-Client Relation," *Yale Law Journal,* 85, 8 (July 1976), 1060–1088. See also Bernard Williams, "Person, Character, and Morality," in Amelie Rorty (ed.), *The Identities of Persons* (Berkeley: University of California Press, 1976), pp. 197–215; and Ferdinand Mount, "Dilution of Fraternity," *Encounter,* 46, 10 (October, 1976), 17–32.

30. MacIntyre, "How Virtues Become Vices..." in Engelhardt and Spicker, *Evaluation and Explanation . . .* , p. 108.

31. MacIntyre is not suggesting or recommending moral relativism. Indeed, he suggests that there are some inescapable moral goods which reflect our social nature, i.e., truthfulness, justice, courage. Moral codes must, in some way, acknowledge the good of truthfulness even if they, in some contexts, allow us to lie to strangers or to great aunts who invite us to admire their new hats. However, MacIntyre goes on to argue that

> the central invariant virtues are never by themselves adequate to constitute a morality. To constitute a morality adequate to guide a human life we need a scheme of the virtues which depends in part on further beliefs, beliefs about the true nature of man and his true end. But about these matters cultures have of course varied and disagreed. . . . The traditional medical virtues are clearly not to be derived in any simple way from the invariant human virtues. To count them as virtues we need to appeal to certain special beliefs about the specific kind of value we place on the preservation of human life, about the special character of the physician-patient relationship and about professional autonomy. The difficulty about the traditional medical virtues is twofold: they have become problematic and they have become problematic in a culture which precisely lacks the means to solve moral problems ("How Virtues Become Vices..." in Engelhardt and Spicker, *Evaluation and Explanation . . .* ," pp. 104, 105).

In my language the invariant virtues require a narrative if they are to be displayed in a manner that can guide our lives. For a position similar to MacIntyre's see my "Natural Law, Tragedy, and Theological Ethics," included in this volume.

32. Alasdair MacIntyre, "Moral Agents in Medicine," in T. H. Engelhardt and Stuart Spicker (eds.), *Philosophical Medical Ethics: Its Nature and Significance* (Dordrecht: D. Reidel Publishing Co., 1977). Mimeograph.

33. Ibid., p. 23.

34. Samuel Gorovitz and Alasdair MacIntyre, "Toward a Theory of Medical Fallibility," in Engelhardt and Callahan, *Science, Ethics, and Medicine,* I, 248–274.

35. Ibid., p. 254.

36. Ibid., p. 255.

37. Ibid., p. 259.

38. Ibid., p. 265. Another important implication of this analysis is how it provides the means to recapture the contribution of the patient to the medical enterprise. The patient is not simply a passive object, but the very willingness of the patients to expose

themselves to risk is a gift to the doctor and other patients. The development of medical skills and experience is dependent on medicine having the cooperation and willingness of patients to participate in the caring process. Medicine thus is not something that doctors practice but rather is an institution that depends on the support of doctors and patients.

39. Eric Cassell, "Error in Medicine," in Engelhardt and Callahan, *Knowledge, Value, and Belief*, II, 20–21. Cassell points out that the new proposals for no-fault malpractice insurance have an interesting implication.

> It might have been suggested earlier that I was wrong in asserting that definitions of responsibility, causality, and injury were relative to the value structure of the group; rather than that, it could be asserted that they were simply relative to our state of knowledge. What was not an injury previously becomes an injury causally related to the action of a responsible physician because knowledge has advanced to reveal the proper action. While that effect of the advance of knowledge is undeniably true, the new "no fault" malpractice proposals suggest that in addition to advance in knowledge, there has also been a change in the group's belief—one should be compensated for injury arising *not only* from the negligence of physicians but also from the action of fate (pp. 16–17).

40. Cassell, "Error in Medicine," in Engelhardt and Callahan, *Knowledge, Value, and Belief*, II, 12.

41. This does not mean that I think it indifferent whether our society uses folk or modern medicine. Generally, I think the ability of modern medicine to cure is impressive and we should be grateful for its power. That does not mean that there are not other ways to conceive of illness and cure that generate a different kind of medicine. But our medicine is "ours" and it is as good and as bad as we deserve. Whether it should be someone else's is up to them.

42. I have argued elsewhere, however, that one of the tasks of the Christian community is to reclaim and form a practice of medicine appropriate to its convictions. While such a task may at first seem self-serving, it is my contention that it is only through such a community's endeavor that all people can have a paradigm for the proper constitution of medicine. Moreover, it is only in this way that we can recover the sense of the importance of traditions and authority for the constitution of medicine as a profession. See my *Vision and Virtue: Essays in Christian Ethical Reflection* (Notre Dame: Fides Press, 1974), pp. 182–186. Even though the force of this essay may appear negative, it is my assumption that there are narratives sufficient to form communities necessary to sustain medicine as a tragic profession. At least I want to claim that Judaism and Christianity embody such narratives.

Index

247

Illich, Ivan, 185–189, 197, 202, 229 n,
239 n, 241 n, 242 n

James, Henry, 76
Jensen, Adolf, 229 n
Jervell, Jacob, 234 n
Jonsen, Albert, 64, 192, 221 n, 223 n,
244 n
Jung, Carl, 227 n

Kamisar, Yale, 230 n
Kant, Immanuel, 47, 50, 54–55, 128,
206 n, 207 n, 208 n, 221 n,
245 n
Kellog, Robert, 76, 224 n
Kiefer, H. E., 211 n
King, Lester, 192, 242 n, 244 n
King, Robert, 244 n
Kluge, Eike-Henner W., 107–108,
229 n
Kohl, Marvin, 228 n
Kovesi, Julius, 21, 207 n, 212 n
Krieg, Robert, 225 n

Ladd, John, 206 n, 241 n, 243 n
Lawrence, D. H., 30
Leech, Clifford, 244 n
Leiser, Burton, 222 n
Lehmann, Paul, 233 n
Lester, Julius, 234 n
Lévi-Strauss, Claude, 229 n
Liberalism, 11, 185, 233 n, 235 n
and community, 10, 196
standard account relation to, 19
political theory of, 205 n
and suicide, 113
interpretation of justice, 141–143,
218 n, 220–221 n
and language of "person," 128–130,
232 n
and tragedy, 241 n
Lifton, Robert, 62, 217 n
Little, 214 n, 219 n
Lögstrup, Knud, 66, 110, 220 n,
229 n
Lonergan, B. F., 225 n
Long, Edward, 215 n

McCabe, Herbert, 64, 219 n
McClendon, James, 80, 214 n, 222 n,
223 n, 225 n
McCormick, Richard, 58, 206 n, 214 n,
223 n, 240 n
McInerny, Ralph, 218 n, 219 n
MacIntyre, Alasdair, 113, 131, 185, 193,
196, 197–200, 201, 202, 204 n,
209 n, 211 n, 222 n, 228 n,
230 n, 232 n, 241 n, 244 n, 245 n
MacKinnon, Edward, 221 n
Mackey, J. P., 215 n
MacPherson, C. B., 205 n
Malcolm X, 97, 227 n
Malits, Elena, ix
Malloy, Ed, 213 n, 223 n
Mandelbaum, Maurice, 43
Marty, Martin, 213 n
Marx, Karl, 21, 208 n
May, William, 156
Mayeroff, Milton, 155, 236 n
Mead, G. H., 161
Medicine, 7, 37, 186, 170–172, 200–
201, 209 n, 242 n, 246 n
ethics of, 8, 20, 168, 184–199, 203 n,
222 n
and "person," 127–131
Melden, A. I., 212 n
Mink, Lew, 75, 223 n, 224 n, 225 n
Moltmann, Jurgen, 233 n
Moore, Hal, 240 n
Moore, Wilbert, 242 n
Mount, Ferdinand, 245 n
Munitz, M. K., 211 n
Murdoch, Iris, 208 n, 209 n, 211 n, 213 n
Murphey, Jeffrie, 240 n

Nagel, Thomas, 221 n
Nakhnikian, G., 212 n
Neuhaus, Richard, 122, 231 n
Niebuhr, H. Richard, 7, 203 n, 207 n
Niebuhr, Reinhold, 132, 227 n, 233 n
Nixon, Richard, 77
Norman, Richard, 212 n
Notestein, Frank, 230 n
Nozick, Robert, 205 n, 235 n

Objectivity, moral, 2, 16, 166, 204 n
as narrative dependent, 17